Praise for *101 Things I Wish I Knew Before I Fed My Children*

"Jenny Harkleroad, in *101 Things I Wish I Knew Before I Fed My Children*, provides a readable synthesis of the truth, making correct decision-making easier."-John McDougall, MD, Author, Researcher, Internist, Co-founder of the McDougall Program.

"*101 Things I Wish I Knew Before I Fed My Children* is a highly informative and comprehensive guide joining the ranks of kindred spirits whose books share the common goal of optimizing American's health through whole food plant based nutrition." -Caldwell B. Esselstyn, Jr., M.D., author of *Prevent and Reverse Heart Disease* and Ann Crile Esselstyn, author with Jane Esselstyn of *The Prevent and Reverse Heart Disease Cookbook*.

"Jenny has created a timeless prescription for individuals, families, and children that is filled with irrefutable scientific research validating a whole-food plant based lifestyle, real actionable recommendations that will lovingly move families toward a healthier lifestyle, and clear guidance for improving the health of children that will assure them of living to their full potential unhindered by disease. It is a must in every kitchen!" -Scott Stoll, M.D., Author, Speaker, Olympian, Co-Founder of the Plantrician Project.

"Thousands of people are now enjoying the blessings of a whole food, plant-based diet. These blessings include amazing, delicious foods, better physical health, and even more mental and spiritual clarity. I am one of them! I'm so grateful Jenny Harkleroad has written this book filled with wisdom and insight to bless the lives of individuals and families. In a world of confusion, this book sheds light on many important topics."-Jane Birch, author of *Discovering the Word of Wisdom: Surprising Insights from a Whole Food, Plant-based Perspective* and DiscoveringtheWordofWisdom.com.

101 THINGS I WISH I KNEW
BEFORE I FED MY CHILDREN

101 THINGS I WISH I KNEW BEFORE I FED MY CHILDREN

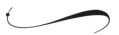

Jenny Harkleroad

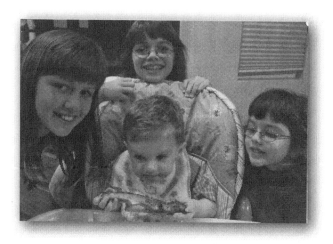

This photo was taken when I thought it was healthy to feed my kids animal protein. Toddler, highchair, and barbecued ribs—why not? I've learned a lot over the years!

Copyright © 2016 Jenny Harkleroad
All rights reserved.

ISBN-13: 9781539039549
ISBN-10: 1539039544

Thank you to my loving husband and our four wonderful children who have been willing to eat for better health. They have also given me time to study health and write about it. I really appreciate their sacrifice. Thank you to my extended family for all your love and support and for eating the plant based foods that I cook for you! Thank you to my best friend Kelli Russell who is always encouraging me to go after my goals and dreams. Kelli taught me to look at things in a way I never did before. She questions things and does not take them at face value. Those lessons have really helped me to learn about health at a deeper level. Plus, a girl needs a best friend and Kelli is that girl for me! Thank you to Alicia Kister for sitting on my bed and teaching me about health when I was too sick to move! Alicia's thoughts sparked my interest in health. So did the results from her advice on choosing better foods. Thank you to Jane Birch, author of Discovering the Word of Wisdom for her wonderful book which helped me understand my religions health code at a whole new level. Thank you also to Jane for her kind heart and willingness to answer my health questions. A big thank you to Dr. John McDougall for his book The Starch Solution, his seminars, recipes, webinars, and the never ending free resources on his website, www.drmcdougall.com. Thank you to Dr. Warren Jacobs who helped me end the unbearable pain I was suffering for years from my broken back. I will be forever grateful to him. Thanks to God for giving me this great opportunity to learn and grow.

Part of the proceeds from this book goes to Operation Underground Railroad (www.OurRescue.org), which rescues kidnapped children from slavery. Nothing breaks my heart like the pain children suffer at the hands of adults. I am in awe of the incredibly hard and heartbreaking but wonderful rescue work you do! Please look up this great non-profit and help to spread the word about them.

DISCLAIMER

ALL INFORMATION CONTAINED in this book and e-book is intended for your general knowledge only and is not a substitute for medical advice or treatment for specific medical conditions. I cannot and do not give you medical advice. If you have any specific questions about any medical matter you should consult your doctor or a qualified professional healthcare provider. If you think you may be suffering from any medical condition you should seek immediate medical attention.

Jenny Harkleroad

TABLE OF CONTENTS

My Story · xv

Chapter 1	The Protein Myth ·	1
Chapter 2	Where Do You Get Your Calcium? · · · · · · · · · · · ·	15
Chapter 3	Are Oils Good for You? · · · · · · · · · · · · · · · · · ·	21
Chapter 4	Eggsposed! ·	27
Chapter 5	Aren't Carbs Evil? ·	33
Chapter 6	Don't Count Calories, Count Health · · · · · · · · · ·	37
Chapter 7	Keep It Simple ·	41
Chapter 8	What Is A Whole Food, Plant Based Diet? · · · · · ·	47
Chapter 9	The Less Ingredients The Better! · · · · · · · · · · · ·	49
Chapter 10	If You Don't Know What An Ingredient Is, Google It! ·	51
Chapter 11	Read The Label! ·	53
Chapter 12	It's Cheaper to Eat Healthy · · · · · · · · · · · · · · · ·	57
Chapter 13	In The Beginning, There Was Food · · · · · · · · · · ·	59
Chapter 14	Pink Salt For Everyone · · · · · · · · · · · · · · · · · · ·	63
Chapter 15	Don't Buy It! ·	65
Chapter 16	Troublemakers ·	67
Chapter 17	Yum! ·	69
Chapter 18	Oh La La! ·	71
Chapter 19	What Is Health Food? · · · · · · · · · · · · · · · · · · ·	75
Chapter 20	Sustainability ·	77
Chapter 21	Vitamins And Supplements · · · · · · · · · · · · · · · ·	79
Chapter 22	Flu Shots And More ·	85

Chapter 23	Water First	87
Chapter 24	The Truth About Americans' Health	89
Chapter 25	The China Study	93
Chapter 26	Veggie Trays On The Table	95
Chapter 27	What To Eat	97
Chapter 28	Antibiotics	99
Chapter 29	What About Pesticides?	103
Chapter 30	Buy Some Kitchen Gadgets	107
Chapter 31	Start Collecting Your Favorite Recipes	109
Chapter 32	Starch For Everyone	111
Chapter 33	Can You Make That?	113
Chapter 34	Sugar Is Not the Enemy	115
Chapter 35	USDA Dietary Guidelines for Americans 2015-2020	121
Chapter 36	Make Your Own Baby Food	125
Chapter 37	Drink Filtered Water	127
Chapter 38	Eat Sprouts!	131
Chapter 39	My Kids Won't Eat That	137
Chapter 40	Food Color	139
Chapter 41	Breastfeeding	141
Chapter 42	Party Like A Whole Food Rock Star!	143
Chapter 43	Brown Bagging It	145
Chapter 44	Make Your Own Birthday Cakes And Frosting	149
Chapter 45	Learn About Grains	153
Chapter 46	Do We Need Portion Control?	155
Chapter 47	Don't Have A "Cheat Day"	157
Chapter 48	Got Ailments?	159
Chapter 49	B12	161
Chapter 50	Human Carnivory	163
Chapter 51	Family Movie Night	165
Chapter 52	Kindness Begins With Me	169
Chapter 53	Don't Do Everything The Doctor Tells You	171
Chapter 54	Switch Your Syrup	173

Chapter 55	Tortilla Chips And Salsa	175
Chapter 56	The Carbohydrate Myth	177
Chapter 57	No More Broken Hearts	179
Chapter 58	Snack On!	183
Chapter 59	Should You Be Gluten Free?	185
Chapter 60	Cashew Cheese, Coconut Yogurt—Yum, But	187
Chapter 61	Nutritional Yeast	189
Chapter 62	Make Your Own Flour	193
Chapter 63	They Will Eat What You Feed Them ... Eventually!	195
Chapter 64	Teach Your Children	199
Chapter 65	Communication	203
Chapter 66	Share The Love	205
Chapter 67	Stripping Greens	207
Chapter 68	If It Has A Face Or A Mom ...	209
Chapter 69	Sweet!	211
Chapter 70	Contradiction	215
Chapter 71	Eat Colorful	217
Chapter 72	Take Care of YOU First	221
Chapter 73	Eat When You Are Hungry	225
Chapter 74	Soaking Whole Grains/Beans/Nuts/Seeds.	229
Chapter 75	Regrow Your Kitchen Veggies/Herbs In Water	231
Chapter 76	To Soy Or Not To Soy?	233
Chapter 77	Got Drugs?	235
Chapter 78	The Glycemic Index	239
Chapter 79	Spice It Up	241
Chapter 80	Eating Animals Is As Bad for You As...	243
Chapter 81	Are Humans Designed To Eat Meat?	245
Chapter 82	The Cure For Acne	251
Chapter 83	Know Your Numbers	253
Chapter 84	Bosom Friend	255
Chapter 85	Unaware	257
Chapter 86	Your Body Absorbed It!	261

Chapter 87	Dry Skin Brushing	267
Chapter 88	Exercise	269
Chapter 89	Mobility	273
Chapter 90	Pop!	275
Chapter 91	Natural Pest Control	277
Chapter 92	Sunshine	285
Chapter 93	Sleep	287
Chapter 94	Find A Hobby	289
Chapter 95	No Mammograms!	293
Chapter 96	Grow A Garden	297
Chapter 97	To Thine Own Self Be True	299
Chapter 98	Skinny	307
Chapter 99	Emotional Eating	311
Chapter 100	Getting Started	319
Chapter 101	Recipes And Cooking Tips	331
	Breakfast	333
	Lunch	335
	Sides, Sauces, And More	339
	Dinner	346
	Dessert	359
	Find Jenny	363
	About the Author	365
	Notes	367

MY STORY

It was 6:15 p.m. on July 4, 2015 and my husband and four kids had just left to enjoy the holiday festivities with friends. So why was I home? That's a long story.

On August 10, 2013, I was in the best shape of my life, thanks to my addiction to Kelli Russell's power yoga classes and being a gym rat in-between them. I was standing on a rock ledge on a mountain in San Diego. I'd been camping and hiking with family and friends, and feeling a little prideful that this easy hike was exhausting some of the people around me. My husband and I got separated from our group and found ourselves standing on a rock, deciding how to get down. My husband Dusty said, "If I was young and in shape I'd jump from here." Well, my pride got the better of me—and I jumped! Really, it did not seem that far. They say it was only nine feet, but I guess that when you land wrong on a rock nine feet down—well, it was enough to break my back! So I started yelling in pain, and vultures started circling (not joking—I wish I was).

911 sent in a ground crew to find me, and then the life flight came. They strapped me down, zip lined me up to a hovering helicopter, and flew me to the nearest hospital. I'm told that I was even on the news. I'm happy to be alive, but the hardest call I had to make that night (actually my husband made the call for me) was to Kelli Russell to let her know I would not be making her Budokon yoga class that night. You now understand my priorities!

Doctors said it would be six weeks until I could go back to yoga. I was not sure I'd survive twenty-four hours, but I could hardly move so that helped to keep me down. It didn't keep the tears from pouring out, though. So, what does a Type A with a very busy life do when bed rest is suddenly non-negotiable? Cry, delete all my yoga classes off my phone schedule, journal, read, find lots of rides for my four kids to their four different schools and activities, get others to help cover my church and volunteer and real estate commitments, and WAIT.

I thought the six weeks would never end, but when they did, I was very aware that my body was not ready for yoga. I wanted to move. I was dying to move. I went to the gym and joined the water aerobics class. It was nice to get out, fun to move, a little odd exercising with grandparents in the pool, and cold, too cold!

After about a month of cold water aerobics, I felt that I could carefully go back to yoga. Boy was that a happy day! Instead of tackling every challenge like I used to, I had to baby every move. Prior to breaking my back, I had a hip injury from doing a cool yoga trick that my body was not flexible enough for. Even though I'd been on bed rest for my back, that hip didn't feel any better. In typical Type A fashion, I did my best to ignore the hip pain. Bad idea! By December 2013 I was starting to limp a bit when I walked because of the left hip pain, and then I had to start missing yoga days. Noooooooooooo!

Another month passed, and I had to stop exercising completely. I could not even walk in a pool as it hurt so much. The doctor ordered an MRI of my hip and lower back (yes, my back was still hurting too) to see what they could find. Unfortunately, they found a round, black circle in my femur bone that sent us on a wild goose chase trying to figure out what it was. First, I was sent to an orthopedic surgeon. He said I was missing part of my femur bone. He said he could do surgery and put screws into my hip to keep it from breaking, but he really didn't know for sure what was going on. The doctor then ordered a bone scan to rule out cancer. Another chain of unfortunate events began.

Apparently I'm allergic to Bone Scan I.V. contrast. This is not the kind of allergy where your heart stops and the doctors attempt to resuscitate you or stick you with an EpiPen®. This was an after the bone scan I'm-not-feeling-well type of allergy. The next day my arms and legs started to tingle. The next day, I couldn't move my legs and went back to the doctor in a wheelchair. The doctor said it might be multiple sclerosis or Guillain–Barré syndrome. Off to the neurologist I went, and then back to the lab for an MRI of the brain to rule out MS. The neurologist stuck me with a bunch of safety pins. Really, there is no higher-tech tool to check my sensitivity? "No MS," they said.

Then my arms stopped working. I was slowly becoming paralyzed. I read about Guillain–Barré syndrome, and apparently your body shuts down until your heart and lungs just stop.

I was lying in bed, and could hear the kids playing downstairs. I was losing the ability to speak and really thought that I was going to die. I decided to call my husband. My cell phone was on the bed right next to me. I couldn't move; I couldn't reach my phone. I struggled and finally got to where I could push the speed dial button. He answered. I tried to speak, and I couldn't. He told me he was almost home. Before I knew it, he was standing by bed with my parents, who happened to be in the neighborhood too. I heard them saying they were going to call 911 or run me to the ER. I whispered a faint "no." They took my pulse, rubbed my head, and talked to me. Then they said that I needed to go to the hospital. Again, I forced out an almost silent "no." For some reason, they listened to me and stayed by my side, taking my pulse, blood pressure (my chiropractor dad happened to have a blood pressure cuff with him) and watching me breathe. Within a few hours, the feeling started coming back into my body and I "woke up." I was able to move a bit and speak. It was as if the allergic reaction had hit its peak and I was on the recovering side of the reaction.

The next morning a lovely friend from church, who is one of those people that is so healthy that you wonder if it's healthy to be that healthy, was sitting on my bed with a basket of health remedies to cure me of this allergic reaction. It was a mix of green powders, herbs, vitamins, lemon, etc. She then spoke to me about health and the body's ability to heal. She cried, and read me our church health code. I was surprised how much health touched her. She inspired my interest, desire, and wonder about health, and put me on a detox that second.

The following week I went to the UCSD Cancer Center to review my bone scan and hip issues. The doctor said they didn't think the dark circle in my hip bone was cancer, but they thought my hip was about to break if I put any pressure on it. If it broke I would need a hip replacement, and they actually considered admitting me right then to do a hip replacement. They took another x-ray though, and decided to hold off. They ordered another MRI and handed me a pair of crutches. How does a mom of four, realtor, and Relief Society President (I ran the women's organization for our congregation, with about two hundred and seventy women in our group of the Church of Jesus Christ of Latter-day Saints, aka Mormons) and helped with other local charities live her life on crutches? Not to mention all the other drama I had recently been through from breaking my back?

I went to the fridge to get some food. How do you open the fridge without letting go of the crutches? How do you do anything with your hands while holding crutches? I strategically placed rolling desk chairs around my house so I could skootch with my good right leg to the fridge, and then to the counter, and over to the blender making my green detox drinks, and from the washer to the dryer, and so on. Later that day, a friend brought a wheelchair and that worked even better. Those swivel wheels on that wheelchair were awesome, and I was back in business!

I went back to the cancer center to review my MRI, and the doctor said "Your left hip ligament is torn really badly. I mean really bad, like you were in a horrific car accident. Your hip was pulled out of the socket very hard during your back breaking landing, and snapped back. It's extremely stretched out and needs four months to heal, but the good news is you don't need the crutches." Happy day! More tears! No cancer, no MS, no hip replacement, no Guillain–Barré, no wheelchair, no crutches. Happy dance (ouch, my hip and back)!

In the meantime, those green drinks were working. I was starting to get some feeling back in my arms and legs! I also started getting curious about green drinks, and my mom introduced me to the Green Smoothie Girl[1] books. I even got to hear one of her lectures in Carlsbad, CA. Of course I stood in the back of the room because my back did not let me sit in a chair.

I was also excited that I had not gained any weight even though I was not going to the gym. Replacing my typical chocolate protein powder breakfast shake which I blended in dairy milk with a green drink was changing my desires of what to eat each day. I went from being a crazy calorie counter to only counting the health I was putting in my mouth. And, my weight didn't change from when I was "the crazy exerciser." It actually started to drop a bit.

Next stop, kinesiologist, body worker, chiropractor, acupuncture, someone fix me up, please! The kinesiologist assigned walking. Ha! Not easy with a torn hip ligament. My goal was to walk out the back door to my fence and back. This was amazingly hard to do, and so painful after I was back inside that I could hardly stand it. Eventually, though, the hip did heal and I got up to walking for about 40 minutes on the treadmill.

As a Type A personality I really, really, really don't like to waste time. There is so much to be done! I know I drive my family a bit crazy with that. They all jump when I come around the corner and try to look productive. Sorry, family. I could not bear to watch TV (wasting time) while on the treadmill.

My mom (thanks mom), introduced me to *Chef Brad's Fusion Grain Cooking Show*.[2] I loved my treadmill time, and used it to take notes on his recipes and cooking methods, which led to adding more grain into our family's diet. I was really excited because the Mormon health code, which is called the Word of Wisdom,[3] in addition to many other things, says to eat meat sparingly and I was doing the opposite. I was caught up in the high protein diets of the day, eating a lot of chicken and veggies and avoiding carbohydrates like grains. I started using half the amount of meat in our meals and adding grains to my recipes instead. It was yummy and healthy, and my family only complained a little.

Did I say I was walking 40 minutes on the treadmill each day? Actually 40 minutes was my maximum. It's like when you are on a diet and you hit your goal weight and never see that number again. Forty minutes on the treadmill turned to 30 minutes, and then to 20, then to 10, and then to "My back hurts so badly. Why?"

By December 2015, I was having more x-rays and thinking that I might have to have back surgery as all my holistic methods were not giving me enough pain relief to live my life or even sit in a chair.

In January 2015, I called to make an appointment with a surgeon; the first opening they had was April 22, 2015. I decide to wait, as I really wanted to see the *best* surgeon, not just any surgeon. By the end of January I was not sure I could survive until April, and I dug out all the old painkillers they had given me in the hospital when I first broke my back. I'm not a big fan of medication, and I figured if I could deal with the pain without it I would. I had reached the I-can't-deal-with-it spot. The problem is that I'm very sensitive to medication and those pain killers just put me to sleep. I actually slept for the entire month of February 2015. Luckily, my body got used to them, somehow, just in time for me to wake up for the crazy hot real estate market that started in March.

I called the surgeon's office, begging them to get me in sooner, and they snuck me in the back door by seeing the surgeon's PA. Of course when I saw her, what did she want? New x-rays, new MRI, CAT scan, bone density test, blood tests, pain doctor for pain injections and more pain pills, etc. So my husband, mom, and friends drove me to all these appointments as I lay in the back of the car because it hurt too much to sit up. It was really embarrassing though, because when I get frustrated I cry; and boy was I frustrated! I wanted to be out of pain and wanted my life back! So, every doctor got to see the sobbing, crazy lady act, which was embarrassing, but all I could do. Unfortunately, the surgeon was concerned that my pain was lower than the broken spot and was not sure that the surgery would help. He asked me to get other opinions. I saw two more surgeons and they said the same thing, but with a bit more confidence that surgery would fix my pain.

In the meantime, I had about ten escrows in process in my real estate career, and decided to have surgery with the third surgeon I saw. I needed to wait for some real estate work to finish, so I scheduled the surgery for May 18, 2015, the Monday after eight of the ten escrows had closed. I got my business partner, Brenda, to cover for me after that.

Surgery went well, minus a lung puncture that was not in the plan. The surgeon fused the L2-L3 vertebrae and replaced the disk with a synthetic one. I was stitched up in six different places on my back and side seven hours later. Recovery was pretty tough! I remember them saying that I had to sit up in the hospital the first day after surgery. Sitting sounded like an impossible task as my body felt so beat up and really unmovable. Before I knew it, I was sitting up, then walking with a walker and headed back home to recover.

As time passed, my interest in health grew. Before my surgery I did the GreenSmoothieGirl twenty six-day detox, which is vegan. When the detox was done, the thought of meat really turned my stomach and I started cooking with grains and starches like potatoes, beans, corn, and sweet potatoes instead of meat. My family was not too happy, so every once in a while, I'd add a small amount of meat to dinner, but it just seemed gross to me, making a delicious dinner and then adding some chopped up animals in it. Nasty! I really can't believe there was a time when I ate meat at almost every meal. My body didn't crave meat anymore, and my brain and mouth were totally repulsed by it.

During my recovery from back surgery I decided that I wanted to read more health books and study my religious health code at a deeper level. Most people know that Mormons don't smoke, use tobacco, drink alcohol, coffee or tea, or use illicit drugs, but did you know we are encouraged to only eat meat in times of winter, cold, or famine and better not to eat meat at all? Mormons are also instructed that grains are to be the staff of life and to eat fruits and herbs. We are promised great blessings of health and knowledge by following this law. As time has passed I see that I am still reaping so many blessing by following this recommendation of not eating meat even though it's not mandatory. I feel so blessed and thankful!

JENNY HARKLEROAD

After studying this religious health code and many health books, including *The China Study, Whole, Discovering the Word of Wisdom, Prevent and Reverse Heart Disease, The Starch Solution, Comfortably Unaware*, and many more (plus much of my own personal experiences with health and diet), I really wanted to share what I had learned. My kids were already half grown when I learned the real truth about health. Not little like they are on the book cover. I am very grateful for my family who are understanding and open-minded about what I have recently learned about health and have not complained too much about all the changes in the kitchen. They are learning and sharing this information with others too, which really warms my heart!

Here are 101 health tips I wish I knew when I got married and started feeding my family. My hope is that this list will not overwhelm you, but that it will give you ideas. Pick one thing you can change today, and maybe another next week. Make a commitment to yourself to learn about health. We have been blessed with these amazingly complex bodies that even scientists don't fully understand. We need to take care of them so that we can live in health and happiness, be in tune with God and fill the measure of our creation.

The first five chapters are the most urgent for turning your health around. If you don't want to deal with 101, just do five. If you do want to do 101, don't get sidetracked and lose sight of the five! Back to the basics will get you healthy.

CHAPTER 1

THE PROTEIN MYTH

YOU NEED MEAT for protein. False! You don't need as much protein as you think and you don't need it from animal products. That might come as new information to you; I know it did to me. How are we supposed to know that we don't need animal protein when the government, schools and even my *Boy Scout Den Leader Manual* are telling us that we need at least 25% protein on our plate at each meal? The other recommended categories of food are vegetables, fruits and grains and a large side of dairy. What are we supposed to think goes in the 25% protein section? Meat! That's what the meat industry is telling and selling us, but it's not the truth. People who make money selling meat want us to believe that the more meat we eat, the better. We Americans love our meat, so we happily go along with this false information. I think the saying should be changed to "As American as apple pie and hamburgers and hot dogs!" Not only do we like meat, we think it's good for us. We think it keeps us slimmer and healthier than if we didn't eat it. But are we healthy?

In *The China Study*,[4] the largest nutritional study ever conducted on the effects of animal protein on disease, Dr. T. Colin Campbell teaches us the surprising truth about what really causes disease. It's no mystery. We can stop looking for a cure because the cause has been found. That's too good to be true, right? Wrong! Here is the truth he found. Dr. Campbell thought that the solution for the world's hunger and disease was to increase animal protein intake. He was quite astonished when he found out that his family members were dying of cancers and heart disease at young ages when they lived on a farm eating home grown meat and dairy products in large quantities. Dr. Campbell discovered through his studies in China and in his lab at Cornell University that it was actually animal protein that turned on disease, namely cancer, in his studies. Dr. Campbell found that you could turn cancers on and off like a light switch by keeping your animal protein consumption under 5% and turning cancer growth right back on when you increase that percent of intake over 5%. When the animal protein intake was over 20% you have a 100% chance of getting cancer according to his studies. I'm really happy that Dr. Campbell had and still has the courage to find and research these facts for his entire career and then promote a whole food, plant based diet when it was anything but popular in the past, and even now.

Dr. Campbell also reminds us of the number of people suffering from disease in our country and the cost of healthcare compared to our total economy. Campbell says that one of every seven dollars in our economy goes to our healthcare. We spend more money than any other country on healthcare, yet we are ranked as having the 37th best healthcare system.[5] The numbers are staggering.

I learned that heart disease is a "toothless paper tiger" in the book *Prevent and Reverse Heart Disease*.[6] According to the author, Dr. Esselstyn, heart disease does not have to kill or even exist![7] You can eat your way out of heart disease, and Dr. Esselstyn has lots of proof. Esselstyn says that 1 in 2 men and 1 in 3 women in the U.S. have some form of heart disease, and we spend 250 billion dollars per year treating the symptoms of that disease when it need not exist at all. This was very exciting news for me as heart disease runs in my family. I could now prevent this disease!

I recently met an adult missionary couple who just got back from serving in Uganda, and she said that heart disease is pretty much non-existent in that country. She says it's due to their diet of starches, fruits, and vegetables. Although I've heard that before, and believe the studies, it's great to meet someone who has been to Uganda and has seen the health first hand of those not eating much animal protein.

Dr. Campbell also reminds us that cancer is not a naturally occurring event. The American Cancer Society[8] states that about 1,685,210 new cancer cases ("this estimate does not include carcinoma in situ (noninvasive cancer) of any site except urinary bladder, nor does it include basal cell or squamous cell skin cancers, which are not required to be reported to cancer registries")[9] are expected to be diagnosed in 2016 in the U.S. In 2016, about 595,690 Americans are expected to die of cancer, or about 1,632 people per day.[10] Last year, the number was 1,620[11] deaths per day. An estimated 10,380 new cases of cancer are expected to occur among children 0 to 14 years of age in 2016 in the US.

Why, when we are spending so much money on a cure, is this disease happening more and more? It's the food we are putting in our bodies, pure and simple. Dr. Campbell proved in his book *The China Study* that he could turn cancer on and off by decreasing animal protein intake under 5%. If this is true, and it is, why don't we try it and see what happens to the cancer numbers in America? If you poison yourself for your whole life by eating foods that you were never biologically designed to eat in mass quantities, you will develop disease. Some people have weaker constitutions and develop disease when they are young. For others, it takes a lifetime of abuse. We can fix this!

We hear that less people die from cancer with early detection, but that is because they find the cancer before it has a chance to make you sick. That sounds good, but is it? After finding cancer, your healthcare professional treats you with drugs and/or surgery and radiation in an attempt to kill the cancer. Have you ever considered that the cancer they found may never have bothered you or made you sick in your entire life? During and after treatment, you suffer both mentally and physically, as does your family. You may possibly drain your life savings trying to save yourself when you were not even sick to start with. Hey, but you're still alive, right? Of course you are. You were fine when they found a cancer and you're still fine. Did they really "save" you? It's something to think seriously about. We have so much faith in doctors and do whatever they say, but they are only trained in treating disease, not prevention or reversing disease, which is an option we can choose.

Americans also suffer from diabetes, which 1 in 13 Americans have, and that number is growing rapidly.[12] From 1990-1998 the rate of diabetes went up 70% in 30 to 39-year-olds. WOW! Have you ever been around someone with diabetes? It's a pretty miserable way to live, especially when you know that it can be prevented or reversed. I'm talking about Type 2 diabetes here. I know people who have died from diabetes, gone blind, had limbs removed, and more. Not to mention the blood sugar checking and monitoring and even dialysis. These diseases are not normal or natural; but we accept them and suffer when most of our suffering can be avoided with proper diet alone. Did you know that you can cure Type 2 diabetes in 10 days on a plant based diet? Why doesn't everyone know that? The truth is right before our very eyes! If you'd like to listen to a very detailed lecture on diabetes, check out this free lecture by Dr. John McDougall, entitled *"Diabetes, Drugs and 100 Years of Missed Opportunities[13],"* at https://www.drmcdougall.com/health/education/videos/free-electures/diet-drugs-and-diabetes/.

The third leading cause of death in the U.S. is death by medical treatment.[14] That's right, we die from surgeries, drugs we are prescribed, and treatments by doctors trying to help us battle our diseases of affluence. Instead of all this disease and cost and suffering, we could do something easy—change what we put in our mouths.

We now have archaeological proof than people have been eating starches as their main source of food as far back at 105,000[15] years ago, and this was happening all over the world from warm to cold climates. These findings are contrary to what we've heard about people consuming mostly animal foods, especially in Paleolithic times.

Let's go back 10,000[16] years. Thanks again to archaeological research; we've learned that North, Central and South America have been eating corn for 7,000 years. People in South America also ate potatoes for 13,000 years. America, Asia and Europe have been eating legumes[17] (alfalfa, clover, peas, beans, lentils, lupines, mesquite, carob, soybeans, peanuts and tamarind) for 6,000 years.

People in South America and the Caribbean ate sweet potatoes for 5,000 years. Africans ate millet for 6,000 years and East Africans ate sorghum for 6,000 years. Middle Easterners ate barley and oats for 11,000 years, people of the Near East ate wheat for 10,000 years and Asians ate rye for 5,000 years and rice for 10,000 years.

Not only does archaeology prove our diet of the past, so does our DNA, and our biology, too.[18] Our DNA is closest to chimpanzees', who are almost purely vegetarian. One thing that is different in our digestive genes is that we have six to eight times more amylase than chimpanzees. Amylase is an enzyme that breaks starch down into simple sugars. Not only do our bodies work best on starches, but we love them. They are satisfying, nutritious and delicious.

We've been lead to believe that we need lots of protein each day and that the best protein is from animals. There are many reasons for this belief.[19] Scientists like Carl Voit[20] believe in protein, and although he found that humans need 48.5 grams per day he recommended 118 grams each day, because he thought you could not get too much of a good thing. 1 gram = 0.00220462 of a pound. If you multiply 48.5 grams (the amount of protein needed per day) x 0.00220462 (1 gram converted to pounds) that gives you 0.1069231 pounds of protein per day that your body needs. So you need about one tenth of a pound of protein per day. That is not much protein, and that amount can easily be obtained from starches, including grains, fruits and vegetables.

Can you understand how you could cause your body harm by eating slabs of meat when your body only needs one tenth of one pound of protein per day to function properly? It's like filling parts of your car engine that don't need it with oil. It causes major issues! Also, it's not animal protein we need but plant protein.

Scientist Voit went on to mentor several scientists of his day, passing on his belief in high protein intake. One of those protégés of the early 1900's was W.O. Atwater, who became the director of the United States

Department of Agriculture (USDA). He recommended 125 grams of protein per day, but 55 grams is recommended now or about .1212541 of a pound of protein per day.

Protein is a buzz word in our society. But how much do you really need? Americans in general eat 75% more protein per day than their bodies need. Try to keep your protein intake to what your body needs. Otherwise, you overtax your kidneys, which are trying to process all that unneeded protein that your body can't store but has to eliminate.

Did you know that you can get all your protein from plants? Here are some examples of the amount of protein in plant based foods, starting with grains and beans. One cup of oats[21] (raw) has 26.3 grams of protein per cup; spelt, our family's favorite grain, has 10.7 grams of protein per cup. Quinoa (pronounced keen-wa) is a popular grain that has 8.1 grams of protein per cup. One cup of rye grain has 17.5 grams of protein, one cup of corn has 15.6 grams of protein, one cup of cooked brown rice has 5 grams of protein, one cup of cooked whole wheat pasta has 7.5 grams of protein per cup, one cup of cooked oatmeal has 5.9 grams of protein, one cup of cooked wild rice has 6.5 grams of protein. One cup of boiled soybeans[22] has 28.6 grams of protein (we ate these last night—yum!), one cup of cooked lentils has 17.9 grams of protein, one cup of cooked white beans has 17.4 grams of protein, one cup of cooked black beans has 15.2 grams of protein, one cup of cooked pinto beans has 15.4 grams of protein.

One cup of spinach[23] has 5.3 grams of protein, one cup of squash has 5.1 grams of protein, one cup of banana[24] has 1.3 grams of protein, one cup of strawberries has 1.1 gram of protein, and a peach has 1.4 grams of protein. One wedge of watermelon has 1.7 grams of protein, and one cup of blackberries has 2 grams of protein.

You can see that there is plenty of protein in plant foods. You don't need to track your protein consumption, even on a plant based diet. Eat a diet heavy in starches like grains, potatoes, corn, legumes, and sweet potatoes and you will be full of energy, strength, health and protein.

Another misconception is the term "high quality protein.[25]" Meats and dairy and eggs are considered to be high quality protein as they easily convert to the protein our body needs. "Low quality" protein comes from plants and converts more slowly to the protein our body needs. Because of the terms high and low quality, and without looking into it further, you could easily think that "high quality protein" would be best for your body but that is not the case. Your body is made to take your food and break it down into what it needs to operate. There is no benefit to eating high quality protein, and lots of detriment.

You can build muscle without eating meat. *Mr. Universe 2014, Barny Du Plessis announced in a recent interview that he's now "all about the vegan gains." Soon after winning the Mr. Universe contest, Du Plessis transitioned to being a "one-hundred percent, wholehearted, staunch warrior vegan." Since going vegan, he has actually gained even more mass; now at 107 kilos or 240 lbs., he claims that there's been no negatives. He wakes up with more energy and recovers faster. This is quite an endorsement for the vegan lifestyle from someone who takes his physique very seriously. Barney is not the first bodybuilder to make waves by being a devoted vegan– just check out PlantBuilt.com—but he is the 2014 Mr. Universe, which puts him in a unique position to help combat common myths about eating vegan. "If you have a good variety of different food like beans, nuts, pulses (dry beans like pinto beans, kidney beans and navy beans; dry peas; lentils; and others), grains, rice they all have protein in them." As for the haters, he exclaims, "People say you can't be a top athlete as a vegan. Absolute bullocks!*[26]

Two years after going vegan, Germany's Strongest Man, Patrik Baboumian, demonstrated that a plant-based diet had not diminished his phenomenal strength or physical performance. In the fall of 2013, Baboumian set a world record for heaviest weight carried a distance of 10 meters, shouldering a yoke weighing more than 1200 pounds (550 kg). Baboumian said, "It's a bit stupid to do things like that, it really hurts," but added that he wants to disprove the myth that anyone, including athletes and strength performers, needs animal products to excel.[27]"

Baboumian has great concern for animals too. He says, "Strength must build up, not destroy. It should outdo itself, not others who are weaker. Used without responsibility, it causes nothing but harm and death. I can lift the heaviest weights, but I cannot take the responsibility off my shoulders. Because the way we use our strength defines our fate. What traces will I leave on my path into the future? Do we really have to kill in order to live? My true strength lies in not seeing weakness as weakness. My strength needs no victims. My strength is my compassion." This is a message to all those out there who think that you need animal products to be fit and strong. Almost two years after becoming vegan I am stronger than ever before and I am still improving day by day. Don't listen to those self-proclaimed nutrition gurus and the supplement industry trying to tell you that you need meat, eggs and dairy to get enough protein. There are plenty of plant-based protein sources and your body is going to thank you for stopping feeding it with dead-food. Go vegan and feel the power![28]

Social psychologist Melanie Joy writes, "Becoming aware of the intense suffering of billions of animals and of our own participation in that suffering can bring up painful emotions: sorrow and grief for the animals; anger at the injustice and deception of the system; despair at the enormity of the problem; fear that trusted authorities and institutions are, in fact, untrustworthy; and guilt for having contributed to the problem. Bearing witness means choosing to suffer. Indeed, empathy is literally 'feeling with.' Choosing to suffer is particularly difficult in a culture that is addicted to comfort — a culture that teaches that pain should be avoided whenever possible and that ignorance is bliss. We can reduce our resistance to witnessing by valuing authenticity over personal pleasure and integration over ignorance.[29]"

My husband recently went on a four-mile hike with our son and his scout troop. My husband and son had potatoes for breakfast. Most of the other scouts had eggs, sausage and bacon. My husband observed that he and my son completed the hike with vigor, but some of the others, especially one boy in particular, were really struggling to complete the hike. My husband ended up going and finding this young man's parents to help him complete the hike. It is hard for our bodies to perform when we give them the wrong fuel.

More in the past than now, protein was connected with status. While almost all classes of people in America can afford animal protein today, this was not always the case. Only the rich ate meat in our country's recent past. Who wanted to feel that they were poor and unable to afford meat? No one, of course, so eating meat proved your social status. Ask any of the older generation and they probably remember this social status. They were the ones who wanted to provide meat to their families, and did so way too well.

Most of us in America grew up eating meat, and that is what we've developed a taste for. We've also been convinced it's healthy. This reminds me of the story of the ham. A new bride was cooking a ham and chopped off both ends before putting it in the oven to roast. The groom asked why she did that, and she said, because that is how her mom did it. She called her mom and asked why she chopped both ends off the ham before cooking it. Mom said, "that's how grandma did it." Grandma was called, and reported that her pan was too small.

We have a meat eating epidemic, and we have a health epidemic, and we have proof that animal protein causes disease. Do we keep eating our animal protein and keep getting disease, or do we change our ways? The choice is up to us. If we are parents, I think we have a responsibility to teach our kids the truth and give them the best chance for good health that we can.

Start thinking about getting your protein from plants. For me, it was really amazing that I could eat carbs, aka starches, and not gain weight. Hadn't I tried that in the past and gained weight? Yes! So what is the difference now? The difference is I'm eating starches with no added oil or dairy or animal products so the calories are low and the healthiness is high. I'm feeding my body what it was designed to run on—whole plant foods.[30]

I've learned that our bodies are made to run on sugar! No, I didn't say go "grab a soda." I'm talking about glucose. When you don't feed your body glucose it runs out of its stores in less than one day, and you actually become sick. Not sick like having a cold or flu, but sick as in your body does not have the nutrients it needs to function properly.

Ever heard of ketosis? You might even think ketosis is good. Living off your fat stores sounds great, right? Well, not really. Ketosis actually mimics sickness. Your body goes into a state of starvation which forces it to live off your fat in order to survive. Most people on this type of diet feel sick and even lethargic and usually lose their appetite. Of course calories are reduced since three-quarters of the dieter's past diet can no longer be eaten. The thrill of quick weight loss can keep some people going. When you stop eating glucose your body empties its water reserve almost immediately, which means you could lose up to three pounds the first day. Don't be fooled by diets that actually make you sick to induce weight loss. Once you stop making yourself sick to lose weight, what happens? Here comes the weight, back again. These diets also cause heart disease, cancer, diabetes, and osteoporosis, to name a few health problems, because all the foods you are eating are poisons.[31]

15 reasons why you may want to reconsider eating meat:

1. *Meat is very high in fat, especially saturated fat.*
2. *Meat is very high in cholesterol.*
3. *Meat is very dense in calories.*
4. *Meat produces carcinogenic compounds when cooked.*
5. *Meat increases chances of colon cancer.*
6. *Meat is hard on the digestive system.*
7. *Meat carries the highest risk of bacterial contamination.*
8. *Meat increases chances of autoimmune diseases.*
9. *Meat contains synthetic hormones, which disturb our hormonal balance.*
10. *Meat contains various drugs.*
11. *Meat contains its own diseases.*
12. *Meat eating results in killing billions of animals each year.*

13. Meat production leads to wasted natural resources like water and land.
14. Meat production is heavily responsible for climate change.
15. Meat raised under stressful conditions has a negatively altered biochemistry, that negatively alters ours.[32]"

When eating a whole food, plant based diet your body gets everything it needs to be healthy and strong and avoid disease, with the exception of vitamin B12, which you can get by taking a B12 tablet, and Vitamin D, which you can get by spending some time in the sun each day. See my B12 chapter for more details. Some people say that the need for B12 proves that we need meat. The problem is that while a little meat may be okay (less than 5% of your diet), we Americans do things on a big scale, and we are much more likely to find good health avoiding meat completely and taking a B12 supplement if needed then we are to try to eat meat sparingly and failing miserably. Don't forget that B12 is really a bacteria, not a vitamin. B12 stays in your system for a long time.[33]

The meat companies in America are happy to spend $100+ million per year promoting a lot of false information about why we need meat for our health. The truth is that Americans are getting about 75% more protein than they need daily, which leads to cancers, obesity, heart disease, diabetes and the overtaxing of many organs like the liver.

What else is bad about meat besides the meat itself? What's in that meat? In order for meat companies to make more money, they do everything they can to produce as many animals as possible in as little space as possible, which causes disease in the animals. They treat animals with antibiotics. Even banned antibiotics are found in your meat.[34] Of course you can buy organic, hormone free meat but the animal protein is still a bigger problem than the antibiotics. Eating animals that are filled with antibiotics does have its own set of issues, such as antibiotic resistant infections that kill 23,000[35] American's per year.

Dr. Esselstyn, the author of *Prevent and Reverse Heart Disease*,[36] found that a plant based diet can also cure and reverse even hard to treat cases of heart disease. Once I found this information I started looking for more and was shocked to find how many books and doctors promote this way of life.

Why had I not heard of this sooner? The reason is that the meat and dairy and egg industries spends hundreds of millions of dollars per year promoting the opposite; so everywhere I turn I hear their message, which is, sadly, very far from the truth. Most of America believes it, eats it, and dies from it.

Do any of us not know someone with cancer right now? I literally get the chills when I hear the word "chemo." I know kids, teens, twenty year-olds, middle-aged and elderly people with cancer right now. I can say that I know five to ten people at any given time with cancer, and have lost friends to cancer, too. We don't have to suffer like this, and we don't have to spend money looking for the cure because we know the cause. As Dr. McDougall always says, "it's the food!"[37]

We can prevent disease in ourselves and share what we know. We don't have to suffer and die of modern diseases. It's really our choice. It's so important to share what we know with our families. As a mother, all I want for my kids is their happiness. I teach them everything I can that will help them to be happy throughout their lives, and beyond, because I believe in eternity. Growing up and being addicted to the standard American diet is not happiness. It's obesity, acne, body odor, bullying and disease. Sure it tastes great, but it comes with a huge price. That is not what I want for my kids when they are young, middle-aged or old. It's hard to eat a whole food, plant based diet when surrounded by Oreos®, burgers, fries and milkshakes. Now that you understand the consequences, you can decide for yourself what grade of fuel you put in your body.

Some peoples' bodies do not show signs of abuse as easily as others. Sometimes we think those people are blessed because they can eat whatever they want and not gain a pound. The trouble is, there are plenty of thin people walking around with disease. So even if weight or other health troubles don't bother you yet, don't use that as an excuse to abuse your body. Learn what will make your body thrive now and in the future and stick with that model. We've all heard someone say, "my dad lived to be 99 eating donuts and bacon every day and never even had a cold." The problem is, we don't know if we are like that dad or like a young kid who will get cancer. I hope we will choose to err on the side of health and not test our bodies to the limit to find their breaking point. Maybe the people who are really blessed are those, like me, whose bodies react quickly to abuse.

I remember watching an Oprah show once where a guy wanted to divorce his wife because she had gained 20 pounds over their 20-year marriage. Oprah responded that she could gain 20 pounds in a weekend. While that story was very sad regarding the divorce, and maybe Oprah's rebuttal could have been a bit of an exaggeration, change your thought process. If your body responds quickly when you over eat the wrong foods, this is a blessing in disguise. Most Americans are more concerned about how they look on the outside than how they feel or what their health is like on the inside. So consider what you once thought was a curse to be a blessing.

What about compassion? Now that I have stopped eating meat, I am not sure why I did not think of the animals I was causing to suffer by my lack of concern. Why kill another creature so I can eat it when there are plenty of other wonderful and healthier choices available without killing? This never occurred to me before. I'm happy for all the animals I now save on a weekly basis not, to mention the water and land and Earth's resources that I don't use up. Add my husband and four kids to this equation and it makes a difference to our planet and the animals that we save every day.

Dr. Scott Stoll reminds us[38] that in wartimes meat was rationed and sent to the troops as calorie-dense food. Interestingly, disease plummeted when we ate less meat in America. Sadly, the belief became that if we won the war there would be a steak on every plate. After World War II, America went from producing 68 million animals for consumption per year to 132 million animals per year, and guess what happened to disease? You guessed it! It skyrocketed! We now produce

70 billion (not million) animals per year for consumption. By 2030, cancer will be the number one killer and surpassing heart disease as animal protein turns on cancer growth.

Want to see the science? I highly recommend *The China Study*[39] by Dr. T. Colin Campbell, PhD & Thomas M. Campbell II. Dr. T. Colin Campbell was hired by the Chinese government to find out why some counties in China had higher cancer rates than others by up to 100%. Guess what he found? Those counties with a higher incidence of cancer ate more animal protein and you could actually turn cancer on and off like a light switch by cutting consumption of animal protein. Why don't we all know and understand this today? As Dr. Scott Stoll's grandpa told him, "Scottie, it's all about the money and if you think it's not, just remember, it's all about the money."

CHAPTER 2

WHERE DO YOU GET YOUR CALCIUM?

CONTRARY TO WHAT the milk industry has told you with their $100+ million dollar per year advertising budget and movie stars with milk mustaches, cow milk actually pulls calcium out of your bones. The US has the highest rates of osteoporosis in the world. If you drink milk, you are actually peeing your bones into the toilet. Crazy! And according to Dr. T. Colin Campbell, author of *The China Study*, cow milk casein turns on cancer like a light switch. He did not get this information from running just one test, but from decades of testing in the lab and testing people in 65 counties in China.

How can the government nutrition recommendations tell you that you need a large serving of dairy each day when you don't, and it's actually detrimental to your health? How can they lie and hurt our bodies like this? Pure and simple, it's big money and big business and big subsidies. Yes, there is calcium in dairy; but dairy products are acidic, so when you eat or drink them your body reacts in an attempt to neutralize the pH and pulls the calcium out of your bones to accomplish that. This is why Americans who eat and drink the most dairy products have the most osteoporosis.

And where does the dairy industry start their propaganda? You guessed it, in the obstetrics and gynecology (OB/GYN) offices, with posters and magazines and goodie bags; and in the elementary schools, teaching our children about the "healthy" food plate.

JENNY HARKLEROAD

Twelve facts about milk
by Dr. Thomas Campbell, MD[40]

1. *In observational studies both across countries and within single populations, higher dairy intake has been linked to increased risk of prostate cancer.*
2. *Observational cohort studies have shown higher dairy intake is linked to higher ovarian cancer risk.*
3. *Cow's milk protein may play a role in triggering type 1 diabetes through a process called molecular mimicry.*
4. *Across countries, populations that consume more dairy have higher rates of multiple sclerosis.*
5. *In interventional animal experiments and human studies, dairy protein has been shown to increase IGF-1 (Insulin-like Growth Factor-1) levels. Increased levels of IGF-1 has now been implicated in several cancers.*
6. *In interventional animal experiments and human experiments, dairy protein has been shown to promote increased cholesterol levels (in the human studies and animal studies) and atherosclerosis (in the animal studies).*
7. *The primary milk protein (casein) promotes cancer initiated by a carcinogen in experimental animal studies.*
8. *D-galactose has been found to be pro-inflammatory and actually is given to create animal models of aging.*
9. *Higher milk intake is linked to acne.*
10. *Milk intake has been implicated in constipation and ear infections.*
11. *Milk is perhaps the most common self-reported food allergen in the world.*
12. *Much of the world's population cannot adequately digest milk due to lactose intolerance.*

A *number of factors increase bone building in the body:*

- *Exercise is one of the most important factors in maintaining bone health.*

- *Exposure to sunlight allows the body to make the bone-building hormone vitamin D.*
- *Eating a plentiful amount of fruits and vegetables helps to keep calcium in bone.*
- *Consuming calcium from plant-based sources, especially green vegetables and beans, provides one of the building blocks for bone building.*
- *Exercise and a diet moderate in protein will help to protect your bones. People who eat plant-based diets and are active probably have lower calcium needs. However, it is still important to eat calcium-rich foods every day.*[41]

Here is what happened to me when I stopped consuming dairy products. The weird taste in my mouth that I'I had for over 20 years went away. I stopped getting colds frequently. My tummy stopped hurting, and my underarms stopped smelling bad and so did my feet. I was concerned about the aluminum in deodorant but could not seem to get by without an antiperspirant—until I quit dairy.

How much dairy was I eating? Not much, actually! I'd dip my veggies in Ranch dressing and eat a few sprinkles of cheese on my food maybe every other day; and once in a while I'd have a dollop of sour cream. I guess I'd have an occasional ice cream at birthday parties. I was shocked that I got all those benefits mentioned above when I stopped eating dairy. Those were just the side effects that I realized. I'm sure there are many other positive effects that took place inside my body when I stopped consuming dairy products. For example, my chance of breast cancer and other female cancers was greatly reduced. Is it worth giving up ice cream and cheese to avoid cancer? For me, the answer is yes!

Unfortunately, it takes most people decades of eating meat and dairy and eggs before you cause disease in your body. Our bodies are so well made that most people can really take an enormous amount of abuse to their bodies before they form a disease. There would be more motivation to eat well if you got cancer the minute you drank a glass of milk; but it takes years to get your cells to mutate and then another 10 years before you discover the cancer, as it needs time to grow and be detectable. Most people don't find cancer due to symptoms but by screening, meaning looking for problems in your body.

Is looking for problems in our body best for us? I can tell you that doctors accidentally found a mysterious dark spot in my hip that lead us on a wild goose chase to a possible scary diagnosis (the doctors were mentioning cancer and MS and Guillain–Barré syndrome), and expensive and uncomfortable testing, crutches, a wheelchair, and missed work, that ended with an allergic reaction that paralyzed me for about a month. That investigation was not helpful to me, but it did make the doctors some money and kept them busy. Don't buy into the Western food and medical moneymaking empire. If you don't have a health issue, don't go searching for one. The best way to avoid medical problems is to avoid animal products, oils and processed foods.

Stop drinking cow's milk. The only thing that causes tumor growth faster than the casein in milk is processed soy (like soy protein isolate, found in lots of protein bars and processed food, so don't eat that either). Cow milk causes adverse reactions like allergies, eczema, swollen tonsils, delayed speech, cancer and diabetes.

There are so many delicious milks that are not dairy milk! There are nut milks, rice milks and soy milks, all nutritious and delicious. But like all foods, if you are purchasing non-dairy milk, read the label. I noticed that the nut milk I was buying for my kids' cereal had oil in it. I started making my own vanilla cashew milk with no additives. See the recipe section under Breakfast. It's so easy!

The great part about changing your habits is that you honestly don't miss it once you make the switch. I thought I could never eat Mexican food without cheese or sour cream and honestly enjoy it. I don't miss it one bit. And, my tummy never hurts! Not to mention all the long-term issues I am avoiding.

It was in 1982 that the USDA decided to start calling foods by nutrient names instead of food names. I believe this was an effort to confuse us and keep us eating unhealthy products. If they say to eat less saturated fat, do you immediately decide to cut back on your meat intake? But if they said, "eat less meat" or "eat less dairy," etc., that would be bad for those industries, so the USDA doesn't say it that way.

Where do you get your calcium? Calcium supplementation is unnecessary. There is more than adequate calcium in a plant based diet of whole grains, legumes and especially the green leafy vegetables.[42]

The exciting thing about eating a plant based diet is that you don't need to figure out how much calcium or any other nutrient you need and then try to calculate it. I did list the protein content in some foods in Chapter One just to show you that you will not die from lack of protein. You can eat and enjoy a whole food, plant based diet and you will have every nutrient that you need.

CHAPTER 3

ARE OILS GOOD FOR YOU?

I USED TO think oils were good for me. I was quite confused when I started reading that they were not. I questioned what I was learning. Thanks to Jane Birch, author of *Discovering the Word of Wisdom*, who sent me her Google Docs file full of proof that oils like coconut oil and olive oil are NOT good for me. I'd heard so many good things about oils, especially coconut oil and olive oil, that I did not think twice about using them; and I especially used a lot of coconut oil in my baking, replacing all the butter with coconut oil. I was actually adding oils to recipes that didn't even call for it, on purpose, because I thought it was good for my family. Boy was I confused!

It turns out that oil, let's take coconut oil for example, has no protein, no carbs, no vitamins, no minerals and only .2mg of healthy fat per serving, and more saturated fat than lard! These oils really are just processed fat. We do need fat in our diet, but in a 2000 calorie diet we only need about 1/2 teaspoon per day of fat before we start clogging our heart. We don't need oil pulled out of a coconut, olive, avocado or vegetables. We may like oil because it tastes delicious in our food, but we actually damage the endothelial lining of our arteries as we eat it, just like we kill brain cells while eating MSG. We need whole foods so our body can benefit from all the reactions that happen when we eat a food that contains fats, proteins, carbohydrates, vitamins, minerals, fiber, etc.

"The human body does need fat, but we need very little for excellent health. Every plant naturally contains fat (where does the vegetable oil come from, after all?). Since plants contain the right amount of fats for our bodies, adding extra fat in the form of free oils just goes straight to our hips and bellies. Cooking spray labeled as zero calories and fat-free is 100% fat! (the FDA allows companies to round down to zero.) Non-stick cookware, parchment paper and silicone mats can be used effectively in place of cooking spray. Sauté with water instead."[43]

I love that a whole food, plant based diet does not need calculations, graphs, charts, etc. Eat basic and simple plant based foods. Eat as much as you like! And you will be healthy inside and out. It's so simple and so wonderful!

OIL REPLACEMENTS

There are lots of replacements for oil. What you need to use depends on whether you're cooking or baking. For cooking, water works amazingly well. If you want a little more flavor, use some vegetable broth. If you're baking, applesauce seems to be the perfect substitute for oil. For salad dressings, I skip the oil and just use balsamic vinegar. If you want to spice up your salad dressing a little you can add some apple juice to your vinegar along with a little bit of 100% pure organic maple syrup and a little teff grain just for more texture. For Italian food you can skip the oil completely. After you cook pasta, rinse it in hot water to get the starch off and keep it from sticking. Always get fat-free marinara sauce or make your own.

In America we put oil in everything. Oil is fat, and we don't need fat extracted out of plants and put into our food. We need to eat the whole food so it reacts in our body as it was meant to and in the quantity it was meant to. If you see how many things in your pantry have oil in them, you'll be shocked.

Don't we need healthy oils? Yes, we do, but we get enough by eating a plant based diet, and we don't need to add any additional oils to our diet. When we add oil to our diet we are just damaging our arteries and causing weight gain from excess calories that makes us feel bad about our bodies, sluggish from extra weight, and more susceptible to modern disease.

Sixty-five percent of 12 to 14-year-olds in the United States have early signs of cholesterol disease that is damaging their blood vessels.[44] It makes sense when we have people dying of heart attacks every two seconds in America. Fat restricts the artery, which can cause further blockage in the clogged artery wall and even tearing of the cell lining; then a blood clot forms which stops the heart.

Studies have shown that dementia patients have areas of their brain where they've had lots of mini strokes. These strokes are caused from artery blockages.[45] Cutting the animal products and the fats out of your diet will prevent and reverse heart disease where all other modern-day treatments, at best, put a Band-Aid® on the problem for a while.[46]

WHAT ABOUT OMEGA 3 AND OMEGA 6? DON'T WE NEED OIL TO GET THOSE FATS?

Before studying health, I remember thinking that I needed fish oil for a healthy brain. I later learned some reasons why I should not take fish oil or eat fish and why I get all the omegas I needed from a whole food, plant-based diet. Here is what I learned from some of my favorite doctors.

"Omega 3's are essential fatty acids supplied in adequate amounts in people consuming plant based nutrition with plenty of green leafy vegetables. However, 1-2 tablespoons of flax seed meal or chia seeds daily are perfectly acceptable. Avoid flax seed oil."[47]

"DHA status of vegetarians ' the relatively lower intake of linoleic acid and the presence of preformed DHA (fish) in the diet of omnivores explain the relatively higher proportion of DHA in blood and tissue lipids compared with vegetarians. In the absence of convincing evidence for the deleterious effects resulting from the lack of DHA from the diet of vegetarians, it must be concluded that needs for omega-3 fatty acids can be met by dietary ALA (alpha linolenic acid). ALA is made by plants. Your well-meaning friends and family may insist you eat fish in order to get enough of the essential fat DHA for the sake of your brain. The two fatty acids (fats) that are essential for human health are the omega-3 alpha, linolenic acid (18:3n-3; ALA) and the omega-6, linoleic acid (18:2n-6; LA). Only plants can synthesize these two fats. No animal or fish can make these fats, but they can be stored in their bodies. These essential fats are converted in animals, including fish, to longer chain derivatives, such as DHA and EPA. DHA, which stands for docosahexaenoic acid, is a type of fat found abundant in the membranes of the retinas of the eyes and the brain. DHA is naturally found in human breast milk, and preformed dietary sources for adults include fatty fish. The human body has no difficulty converting the plant-derived omega-3 fat, ALA, into DHA or other omega-3 fatty acids, in the liver, thus supplying our needs even during gestation and infancy. With this solid science you can put your friends' worries at ease—as a non-fish-eater you will be just fine. And you'll also avoid all that toxic mercury and help restore our oceans."[48]

"If I must answer the DHA question, I would only say that we can get plenty of that type of chemical from the consumption of the omega-3 fatty acids that are found in certain plants–certain nuts, flaxseed, etc. Indeed, it also is related to a dietary balance of omega-3 to omega-6 fatty acids and this balance can be readily met with a good quality diet of wholesome vegetables, fruits, grains and nuts. Vegans do just fine when eating in this way. Indeed, there are new findings that for those who have even gone only part of the way toward that goal, they live 10 years longer and have much less of the chronic degenerative diseases than those who still consume regular American fare."[49]

More reasons to avoid fish and fish oils:[50]

1) *Fish cause a rise in blood cholesterol levels similar to the rise caused by beef and pork.*

2) *Their highly-acidic animal proteins accelerate calcium loss, contributing to osteoporosis and kidney stones. The addition of 5 ounces of skipjack tuna (34 grams of animal protein) a day increases the loss of calcium from the bones, into the urine, by 23%.*
3) *No dietary fiber or digestible carbohydrates are present in fish—thus having a negative impact on bowel function and physical endurance, like winning a foot race.*
4) *Although omega-3 fats "thin" the blood, preventing thrombus formation (heart attacks); this same anticoagulant activity can increase the risk of bleeding complications from other sources, like a hemorrhagic stroke or an auto accident.*
5) *These good fats have anti-inflammatory properties, which can be beneficial—reducing arthritis pain, for example, as well as deleterious—causing immune suppression, increasing the risk of cancer and infection. Omega-3 fish fats have been demonstrated to induce 10-fold more metastases in number and 1000-fold in volume in an animal model of colon cancer metastasis than does a low-fat diet.*
6) *Fatty fish, commonly recommended salmon for example, is half fat and loaded with calories, adding to one's risk for developing obesity and type-2 diabetes.*
7) *Omega-3 fats inhibit the action of insulin, thereby increasing blood sugar levels and aggravating diabetes.*
8) *Fish-eating prolongs gestation, increasing birth weight, and the possibility of birth injury and increased mortality.*

CHAPTER 4

EGGSPOSED!

WHILE THE MEDIA likes to promote most animal products and buy into the propaganda like most people do, it seems that eggs are "on again, off again" when it comes to your health and the media. However, on a whole food, plant based diet, eggs are always off the list. I love Dr. McDougall and the 40 years of health he's been promoting. He is a doctor and his goal is to make his patients healthy. He's found that a plant based diet gets rid of many modern diseases, so he does all he can to share this information with other doctors and the public. I've learned so much from all the free information on his website as well as his webinars and advanced study weekends. I really appreciate Dr. McDougall and his health food pioneering! He has changed how I eat, forever.

One of the things I appreciate about Dr. McDougall is that he never beats around the bush. He tells it like it is. He also shares all this information for FREE on his website, www.Dr.McDougall.com.[51] In Dr. McDougall's January 2016 newsletter, here is what he has to say about eggs.

The Egg Industry: Exposing a Source of Food Poisoning[52]
In my June 2015 Newsletter[53] *article, "There Are Lies and Damned Lies: Damned Lies Harm the Public and Planet Earth," I expressed my outrage over an "Opinion" piece in the June 23/24, 2015 Journal of the American Medical Association. The article applauded the Dietary Guidelines Advisory Committee's (DGAC) recommendation for the "elimination of dietary cholesterol as a 'nutrient of concern' and the absence of an upper limit on total fat consumption." The*

JAMA article was referring to the updated 2015-2020 Dietary Guidelines for Americans, released in January of 2016. Previous US Dietary Guidelines[54] had recommended that people consume less than 300 mg per day of dietary cholesterol, which is about one large egg.

Appreciable amounts of cholesterol are only found in animal products, from tunas to turkeys. Of all the foods commonly consumed as part of the rich Western diet, eggs contain the highest concentrations of cholesterol: eight times more than beef. Traditionally, in scientific studies on humans, eggs have been used as the source to demonstrate the adverse effects of cholesterol on our health and our heart arteries. For this reason, the egg industry has taken the lead in misleading the public (including physicians) about the harmful effects of eggs, which are poisonous when consumed in the high amounts typical of American diets.

On January 6, 2016 the Physicians Committee for Responsible Medicine (PCRM),[55] myself (Dr. McDougall), and other well-respected California-based physicians filed suit in the US District Court (North District of California) against the United States Department of Agriculture (USDA) and the Department of Health and Human Service (DHHS) over their DGAC's position "that cholesterol is no longer a nutrient of concern for overconsumption."

The DGAC's position is based on a 20-year attempt by the egg industry to change the public's image of eggs as a contributor to American's number one cause of death: coronary heart disease. The DGAC disregarded decades of independent basic research incriminating cholesterol consumption—in other words "eating animals"—in order to accomplish their task. They instead relied on recent research that was orchestrated and funded by the egg and other livestock industries to communicate the innocence of eggs as a major cause of the multiple illnesses that plague millions of Americans.

As a physician, if this position, "that cholesterol is no longer a nutrient of concern for overconsumption," remained in the 2015–2020 Dietary Guidelines for Americans, I would be harmed because these foods high in cholesterol (meat, poultry, eggs, dairy products, and fish) and saturated fat (animal foods, except fish) impair the health of my patients, making it more difficult for me to accomplish my professional objectives and duties as a medical doctor, to keep my patients healthy, and to reverse their dietary diseases, including obesity, heart disease (atherosclerosis), diabetes, inflammatory arthritis, and various intestinal disorders.

Exposing Industries' Dirty Tricks for Four Decades

This will be a hard-fought battle, as the egg industry has deep pockets. According to the American Egg Board Annual 2014 Report, "Both the growth rate for dollar and unit sales were double that of 2013, and USDA is showing the highest per capita consumption in 30 years." The Board spends more than 23 million dollars promoting eggs. No doubt they will set aside a portion of their budget to deal with us. They will play as dirty as necessary to protect their business interests if we do get significant attention. Because I have so far not been able to expose their dishonesty to a threatening level, I have never been confronted by any of the livestock industries.

My 1983 publication **The McDougall Plan**[56] *revealed that the dirty tricks used today to get Americans to eat more eggs began in the late 1970s. I wrote more than three decades ago, "Of the six studies in the medical literature that fail to demonstrate a significant rise in blood cholesterol level with the consumption of whole eggs, three were paid for by the American Egg Board, one by the Missouri Egg Merchandising Council, and one by the Egg Program of the California Department of Agriculture. Support for the sixth paper was not identified."*

The methods used to show no harm from eating cholesterol (animals) are designing beforehand the experiment to get the results you are looking for. To show little or no increase in cholesterol levels from eating eggs, you first saturate your subjects with cholesterol from other sources (meat, etc.). Studies show that once people consume more than 400 to 800 milligrams of cholesterol per day, additional cholesterol has only a minor effect on blood cholesterol levels. Candidates for an experiment are easy to find since the typical American diet is based on a high intake of cholesterol (meat, poultry, dairy, and fish). Study designs can also use improper control subjects and inadequate time periods for the ingested cholesterol to show effects in the blood.

JENNY HARKLEROAD

Notes about Current Research in The "Complaint for Declarative and Injunctive Relief"

In the past two decades, the American Egg Board and the Egg Nutrition Center have become increasingly active in using research to increase demand for eggs. Of the 41 studies on dietary cholesterol included in a 1992 meta-analysis[57] 29% were paid for by industry, mainly the egg industry. Nine years later, in a 2001 meta-analysis,[58] that figure had risen to 41%. Two decades later, in a 2013 review,[59] the figure was 92%. The food industry now dominates research on dietary cholesterol.

The egg industry, through researchers at Tufts (University)/USDA Center, have an overshadowing influence on the DGAC. The Tufts/USDA Center researchers excluded all studies published prior to 2003. Of the 12 studies that they included, eight were funded by the American Egg Board through the Egg Nutrition Center, two were funded by British and Australian egg industry associations, and the eleventh was funded by the fish industry in defense of prawn consumption. In other words, 11 out of the 12 cited studies were designed to arrive at a specific pro-industry result.

Despite their industry-related funding, nearly every cited study showed that eggs or other cholesterol-containing foods had an unfavorable effect on blood cholesterol levels. Nevertheless, John Griffin and Dr. Alice Lichtenstein (egg industry associated DGAC members) concluded that the effect of dietary cholesterol on plasma lipid concentrations "is modest and appears to be limited to population subgroups.

Eggs Are Perfect for Growing Chicks

The egg industry provides a timely example of how money can buy scientific nutritional information that can be detrimental to the public's health. Citizens of the US and other Western countries suffer diseases of over-nutrition. Yet the Dietary Guidelines for Americans focus on getting enough nutrients (nonexistent problems). We do not suffer from protein, calcium, fat, or vitamin deficiencies (scurvy, beriberi, pellagra, etc.). Our problems stem from too much of the foods and nutrients recommended in the Dietary Guidelines for Americans.

The purpose of a hen's egg is to provide all the materials necessary to develop the one cell—created by the joining of a cock's sperm with a hen's ovum—into *a complete chick with feathers, a beak, legs, and a tail. This miraculous growth and development is supported by a one and a half-ounce package of ingredients, the hen's egg, jam-packed with proteins, fats, cholesterol, vitamins and minerals. A result is the hen's egg has been called "one of nature's most nutritious creations."*

Indeed, an egg is the richest of all foods, and far too much of a "good thing" for people. The components of a cooked egg are completely absorbed through our intestines. As a result, this highly concentrated food, recommended by the 2015–2020 Dietary Guidelines for Americans, provides too much cholesterol, fat, and protein for our body to safely process. The penalties are heart disease, obesity, and type-2 diabetes, to name a few epidemic sicknesses from our food."

"Despite the powerful egg industry's best efforts to put a "healthy" spin on egg consumption, eggs contain high levels of cholesterol and may contain carcinogenic retroviruses, heterocyclic amines, toxic pollutants (such as arsenic, perfluorochemicals like PCB, phthalates, flame retardant chemicals, dioxins), and Salmonella. Consuming just one egg per day may significantly shorten our life span, increase the levels of the cancer-promoting growth hormone IGF-1, and increase our risk of heart disease, kidney stones, stroke, type 2 diabetes, gestational diabetes, and some types of cancer (such as pancreatic, breast, and prostate).

Eating a meatless, egg-less, plant-based diet may improve mood, lead to weight loss, lower the risk of cataracts, neurological diseases, food poisoning, heart disease, diabetes, asthma, help reverse rheumatoid arthritis, and may increase lifespan. This may be due in part to the arachidonic acid, cholesterol, sulfuric acid, choline, methionine, and sex hormones in eggs and the relative lack of antioxidant phytonutrients.[60]"

If that's not convincing enough, Google egg production and see how chickens are treated who produce our eggs. Even the free-range chickens don't have the life we might expect. If you won't give up eggs for your health, please do it for the humane treatment of animals.

CHAPTER 5

AREN'T CARBS EVIL?

FALSE! CARBS ARE not evil! Carbohydrates or starches in whole form are the staff of life. "Please pass the rolls!" One of my favorite lines from *Father of the Bride* occurs when Frank had taken some sleeping pills and fell asleep as he was asking someone to "please pass the rolls." I love that movie! What do people say when you tell them you want to lose weight? They say, keep away from the starches, hold off the carbs, lay off the mashed potatoes, etc.

Picture someone in a rural village in China. What is their diet? Most likely, it is rice and vegetables. Are they overweight? No! But they eat tons of rice, even white rice. How can it be that they are so slim? The answer is that carbs are high in energy, satisfaction, fiber, glucose, proteins and everything your body needs to be healthy and strong and energetic and to feel full and satisfied. People get fat on carbs when they eat processed carbs with added animal fats and vegetable fats.

Carbs don't make you fat. Carbs are good and healthy and needed for a healthful diet. The next time you buy bread, look for 100% whole grain bread with no added oil or eggs. Next time you make mashed potatoes don't add any dairy products to them. Use nondairy milk and a bit of salt to season them, or a pinch of nutmeg like my mom uses. Next time you eat pasta, buy whole grain pasta and make sure that your sauce is free of animal products and oils. You will be amazed at how many carbs you can eat while staying fit, trim and healthy and eating tons of whole carbs without the additives!

I know what you are thinking; "but I don't like potatoes without butter or pasta without cheese." The amazing, awesome fact is this:

you actually will like plain, whole foods if you just try it for a while. "A while" might be two to eight weeks, depending on your taste buds and your willingness. Two to eight weeks may seem to be a long time, but if you are a mom, put it in the perspective of being pregnant. It's actually quite short when compared to carrying a baby for 40 weeks and then 18 years-plus of mothering. Remember, this is your health we are talking about. Good things are not always easy, but I know you can do this! Your body will adjust and actually start to appreciate the wonderful, natural tastes of food. Is it worth having a healthy heart and body, and a disease free healthy life, just by giving up a few things that seem important now but won't be once you adjust? I no longer want meat, cheese, sour cream, eggs or even dessert. I'm feeding my body what it was made to run on and it's happy with me and I'm happy too.

I know, the people who died on the Titanic and didn't eat dessert wished they did; and who knows, maybe you'll get hit by a bus tomorrow, so why not live it up now? And your grandpa ate donuts every day until he died, healthy, at age 99. If you compare your chances of getting hit by a bus to your chances of getting heart disease it's 50%, or the chance of getting cancer 30%, or diabetes 8%—and rising each year—not to mention all the day-to-day blood pressure, digestion, arthritis and other problems that people suffer through. It's not worth the risk!

Have you ever heard of the bread, rice or potato diet? Yes, you can quickly lose weight eating carbs if you cut the fat. The great news is that also saves your heart! My favorite thing about carbs is that they are so satisfying. I feel full when I eat them. Think of the science behind them; because they are low fat and low calorie foods you can eat much more of them that you could compared to meat or dairy or processed food. Starches, more commonly known as carbs, literally fill your stomach and makes your body not want any more food, because your stomach is full. Your glucose stores are restored, and that tells your body you have had enough food. Make carbs (starches) the center of your meal. For example, eat whole grains, unrefined flours, egg free pasta, roots, winter squashes and legumes (beans, lentils and peas.)[61]

People have the wrong information about glucose. When we eat, our blood sugar goes up, and that is good. Because of what we've heard about diabetes and the glycemic index, we think it's best to keep our blood sugar low, and that is not true. Think about hypoglycemia, for example. You can die from low blood sugar. When you only eat low glucose foods, you just want dessert because your body is starving for glucose. Feed your body glucose in the form of sweet potatoes, not cheesecake. Again, you might think that you will be missing out, but I can speak from my own experience and countless others, you will not miss the foods that cause disease.

CHAPTER 6

DON'T COUNT CALORIES, COUNT HEALTH

Do you choose a 100 calorie apple or a 100 calorie snack bag of processed chips? Which will help your body to grow and flourish? Which will leave you satisfied and which will leave you teased and hungry and wanting more? Of course, if you are really hungry, how about a grain or starch with veggies on the side, like pasta and an oil free marinara sauce or a baked potato and salad with a fig vinegar for your dressing? Those types of foods are full of nutrition and energy but low on heart damaging fat and low on calories. Compare that with some meat that has high calories, high fat, and high cholesterol, served with a side salad topped with Ranch dressing, full of fat and chemicals. These fats and chemicals damage your body; and when you do that over and over and over, meal after meal after meal, your body can't function properly and disease takes over.

Our bodies have a vibrational frequency and so does our food. The highest vibration or highest energy foods are fruits, veggies, nuts, seeds, sprouts, greens, legumes and grains. The low vibration foods are all processed foods, all animal products which include meat, dairy and eggs, refined sugar, chemical sweeteners, refined flour, coffee, soda, and canned food. Healthy humans have a vibrational frequency of 62-68 MHz. Human cells begin to mutate when they drop below 62 MHz.[62] We wonder why we are full of disease when we are eating foods that drag our bodies down to the point where our cells mutate.

In 2015 I supported a friend by donating to a three-day walk and I was kind of torn; because, to be quite frank, we are killing ourselves. We are looking for a cure but we don't want to stop eating and drinking the poison. We just want to keep all of our toxic habits and stay healthy. It just doesn't work like that. We need to turn our focus to the cause and not the cure. Of course, there is a ton of contradictory information out there on what true health is, so that is one reason I want to share my message of true health with you.

What about genes? Genes load the gun and diet pulls the trigger. Like Dr. Campbell said in *The China Study*, he could literally turn cancer growth on and off by increasing milk protein intake above 5%. I think we like the genes excuse because we can't do anything about it and we use it as our excuse; but from the books I've read and the studies I've seen, we are the ones pulling the trigger.

Maybe, we say "genes" but what that really means is family traditions, or how we eat and exercise. Is the whole family overweight? Why? Is it in their genes or are they overeaters, junk food eaters, emotional eaters or don't like physical activity? Does heart disease run in the family, or do they all have cholesterol over 150 because of what they eat? Dr. Esselstyn says you are heart attack proof if your cholesterol is under 150. It seems like a pretty important goal right? Is it important enough to change how you eat? That's up to you. For me, I've had my fair share of pain and suffering and anything I can do to avoid more pain and suffering in my future, I'm all over it!

I used to be a crazy calorie counter, and it did work well to keep my weight in check, but I was obsessed with every calorie that went into my mouth and it really was no way to live. Now I keep my weight much lower and my health much better by choosing a whole food, plant based diet. I no longer count calories because I don't have to. What a relief! Do we care more about our outside appearance than our health? Clearly, as a whole, the answer is yes. For me, the answer was yes as well. Let's change that. A side effect of being healthy inside is looking healthy on the outside.

After I had my second daughter, I started a diet, and the deal was that I could have dessert once per week. I honestly thought I would die. Luckily I lived, but barely! The things I eat for dessert now are actually healthy yet sweet, like fruit. In the past, fruit was not enough dessert for me. What happened? As I changed what I ate, my body adjusted and my tastes changed. I didn't try to change my tastes; it just happened. Our bodies need glucose in the form of starches. When we don't give our body that fuel, it's craves glucose. Dessert! Now that I give my body plenty of whole grains, beans, corn, potatoes, legumes, and sweet potatoes, my body no longer wants dessert. It's full and satisfied with the correct fuel. Ask anyone who does not have good health and/or have been fighting their weight their whole life and they will tell you that there is nothing more miserable. Let's avoid that now that we know we can! Choose foods for good health, not for calorie count!

CHAPTER 7

KEEP IT SIMPLE

IN 2015, I was listening to a health talk that my husband sent me. It was about the top four foods to eat, the top three foods to never eat, and the four best ways to stay healthy, or something to that effect. I'm really glad I listened, because it made me see how much confusion is out there. The talk made me think that there is so much deceit in the food and health industry that I didn't even know what to do, so I needed to pay someone to advise me, and they would be giving me the wrong information too because they are just as confused. The information they were sharing was highly influenced by the food industry. I was almost paralyzed with too much information that was really not helpful to me, and I didn't know what to do next.

I'm so glad that I've found the truth about how to be healthy and slim. It's cheap and simple and no secret and many, many, many doctors agree with this exact plan. Here it is. You don't need a note pad or anything; it's that simple.

Eat starches (beans, grains, legumes, potatoes, corn, sweet potatoes) plus add some fruits and veggies. Drink water. Get some sun and exercise. Avoid all animal foods, processed foods and oils. Take a B12 supplement once per week. It's that easy to say, and that easy to understand. Don't get caught up in macro and micro nutrients or any really detailed specifics. This diet is so basic and so simple that it almost seems like something is missing, but it's not.

My questions when I started learning about this whole food, plant based diet were, why eat like that and why get my husband and kids to eat like that? The reasons are because you can avoid, prevent and even cure modern disease by eating like this, and you can save the Earth, animals, your waistline and the family budget! You can't beat that!

Keeping it Simple on a Whole Foods Plant-Based Diet [63]
When I tell people how much I enjoy the simplicity of my diet, often they look confused.

"But it's so complicated, there's so much that you don't eat!"

"It must be so difficult to eat out though, right?"

"All those recipes seem so time-consuming. There's nothing simple about making every meal yourself!"

Top Five Tips
While I can understand these statements, and the fact that many people may view a whole foods plant-based diet as an incredibly complicated venture (even the name's not easy to say!), this couldn't be further from the truth. Fundamentally, this is a diet based on fruits, vegetables, grains and legumes. It's that simple. But, due to the massive volume of dietary information- and misinformation- that we are bombarded with each day, it's easy to get caught up in over-complicating our ideas about what we should put in our shopping carts, on our plates, or in our mouths.

For this reason, I'd like to share my top 5 tips for "Keeping it Simple" on a healthy plant-based diet. My hope is that this will benefit those of you currently transitioning to this way of eating, and help experienced plant-based eaters save themselves some time and confusion too.

1. If it's a whole, plant-based food, you can eat it
If it's a whole grain, a legume, a starchy vegetable, a non-starchy vegetable, or a fruit, then it's considered part of a healthy plant-based diet. If it comes from an animal, or contains oils or highly processed and refined ingredients, it's not. It's not really necessary, or beneficial, to spend time researching if quinoa is better for you than brown rice, or which legume is higher in protein, or which fruit has slightly more vitamin C than another. Unless you have specific dietary requirements that require you to avoid things like gluten, wheat, or legumes,

your health will benefit greatly from any variety of foods you choose to eat within these five groups.

More and more diet-related issues continue to attract concern in the plant-based community, including the importance of eating organically, or avoiding GMOs, or consuming a certain amount raw foods each day, or achieving a specific macronutrient ratio. Some wonder if they should shun gluten (even in the absence of an allergy), others fret about whether they should avoid grains, and many spend hundreds of dollars on 'superfoods' with the belief that they are the true key to optimal health. While some of these issues may warrant your attention, don't let them distract or overwhelm you. Many people that are changing to a plant-based diet become so overwhelmed by all these additional 'rules' that they immediately feel like giving up because it's too hard. My advice...stick with the basics: eat whole, minimally processed, plant-based foods that YOU can afford, and that YOU enjoy eating.

2. Fill the majority of your shopping cart with single ingredient foods

The more foods you buy that contain just one ingredient, the less you'll have to worry or think about what you're putting in your mouth. What do I mean by single-ingredient foods? Anything you purchase in the supermarket that is what it is- with nothing else added! A banana, for example, contains just banana; much like a bunch of fresh kale, or a bag of brown rice, or a pack of dry lentils. Even whole wheat pasta generally contains just one ingredient: whole wheat.

Essentially, all fresh fruits and vegetables, whole grains, legumes, nuts, seeds and frozen fruits and vegetables are single-ingredient foods, and they should be taking up the vast majority of space in your shopping cart. Any remaining space can be used for additions necessary to complete meals, such as plant based milks, seasonings, flour-based products like whole grain breads, and condiments that are free of animal products and oils.

3. Make use of convenience items when necessary

In an ideal world, we'd all soak and cook our own legumes, pluck and prep farm fresh vegetables, and bake our own bread from scratch. The reality, however, is that we lead incredibly busy lives nowadays, and many people find it hard to make one home cooked meal a day, let alone prepare all their ingredients from scratch. For this reason, I have found it helpful to have some frozen and canned items on hand for cooking. While some may disagree with me on this, my principle is simple: if having canned beans and frozen prepped veggies is going to help you stick with a whole foods plant-based diet (and stop you from calling for takeout instead) then it's a good thing!

When purchasing these items, however, it's best to follow these guidelines:

- *Frozen (fruits, vegetables):* No added salt, sugar, or oils
- *Canned (legumes, tomato products):* No added salt or oils

Many supermarkets also sell washed and pre-sliced vegetables in the refrigerated section of the produce aisle. This usually includes things like grated carrots, shaved Brussels sprouts, salad mixes, and stir-fry mixes. These items can be a real blessing when you need to cook dinner after a long work day, saving you time on washing, chopping, and cleaning up, too!

4. Eat simple food combinations, rather than relying only on recipes

This might sound contradictory coming from someone that develops new recipes on a weekly basis, but I feel that this is an important point to make. While I love nothing more that rifling through recipe books on my days off to find something delicious to shop and cook for, on busy days I find it easier to rely on basic combinations of foods. Breakfast might be plain oats with fruit; lunch a baked sweet potato with salad greens, and dinner a mix of brown rice and black beans, with steamed spinach on the side. Pick a grain, a legume, a vegetable, or a fruit, and the possibilities are endless. Season these simple combinations with herbs, spices, or your favorite condiments, and you've got flavorful, healthy meals in a matter of minutes.

To make life really simple, I like to batch cook a whole grain, a legume, and a starchy vegetable at the beginning of the week. You can then rotate combinations of these three things in the days following, adding different fruits or vegetables at each meal. While this might sound monotonous to some, remember that many of the world's longest lived populations rely on relatively few dietary staples for the majority of their lives, such as the people of Okinawa on sweet potatoes, and the locals of Nicoya, Costa Rica on rice and beans. Variety may be the spice of life, but simplicity may just help you live longer!

5. Don't make separate meals for everyone
This is a tip for those with families, and it's something that I've learned from experience. If you're going to go to the effort of preparing a family dinner, plan it so that you don't end up cooking two or three or four separate meals to suit everyone. This is to help preserve your sanity! While I'm very understanding of parents with picky kids, or those with partners who aren't so enthusiastic about plant based eating, things will start to get really complicated if you try to cater to each person individually. In fact, it can make you feel as though a plant based diet is more trouble than it's worth. It's for this reason that I suggest choosing meals that suit (or can be tailored to suit) everyone, at least when you are all eating together.

If you're looking for ideas, things like tacos or baked potato stations are great. You can serve a number of different fillings and toppings and let everyone customize their meal to their liking. Pasta dishes are usually great crowd-pleasers, as are veggie burgers and oven-baked fries. Talk to your family about what meals they like best, and keep them on rotation, changing the vegetables or seasonings used to keep things interesting.

I do hope that some of this information was useful to you! At the end of the day, how you approach a whole foods plant-based diet will depend largely on your lifestyle. And if you're like me—busy, on the go, but still trying to keep yourself and your family healthy—then you'll want to keep it as simple as possible. Find a rhythm, eat foods you enjoy, and don't sweat the small stuff.

CHAPTER 8

WHAT IS A WHOLE FOOD, PLANT BASED DIET?

I REALLY LIKE the explanation in Dr. McDougall's online color picture book because it keeps a whole food, plant based diet simple. https://www.drmcdougall.com/wp/wp-content/uploads/Dr.-McDougalls-Color-Picture-Book1.pdf.[64] If you can't click the link now, here is my summary. Make starches/grains your main food: beans, corn, potatoes, rice, grains (whole grains where possible) and legumes. Eat some fruit, eat some veggies. Don't eat meat, cheese, milk, eggs, or fake animal products. Don't eat oils or processed food. Eat nuts, dried fruit, and avocados sparingly. Take a B12 supplement (see more in Chapter 49 on B12). Get some sun and exercise.

Why eat like this? Because it saves you from disease and it saves the Earth. How, you ask? A whole food, plant based diet saves you from disease because you are not filling your body with processed foods that are full of toxic chemicals, and fat, meat and dairy that increase your cholesterol, which damages the endothelial lining of your arteries. Dr. Colin Campbell proved that milk casein causes cancer growth[65] in the largest nutrition study ever done in the world. It has also been proven that milk causes osteoporosis,[66] which is the opposite of what the milk industry tells you. America has the highest consumption rates of milk and the highest rates of osteoporosis. Processed soy causes cancer growth as well.[67] Also, your liver and kidneys are damaged when you eat too much protein; and the average American eats way too much protein, like 75% too much. Why? We actually think we need lots of protein, although that has been proved to be untrue. We think olive oil is good for us, but it's just a processed fat that has been found to be no better than animal fat consumption.[68]

How does the toxic American diet ruin the earth? It's because of the resources required for the foods that are part of the diet. We use a lot of food and water and land and energy to produce meat and dairy. It takes 1.5 acres of land to produce 37,000 lbs. of plant food or 375 lbs. of meat. In other words, to feed one vegan for one year it takes 1/6th of an acre. To feed one meat eater it takes 18 times as much land than is needed for one vegan.[69] When the cost of starches goes up and there is not enough to go around, and not enough at a low enough cost to feed the world's poor, people starve so we can eat animals. That's a pretty eye opening statement, don't you think?

During the mid-1980's famine, Ethiopia was a net exporter of food. The government and businesses exported food to be used as feed to produce meat and other animal-based foods for wealthier countries and individuals.

Those with greater financial resources bid food away from those who have less because they're able to pay higher prices. It's hard to believe but exporting large quantities of food is a common practice that continues today in Ethiopia, Kenya and other countries with large populations of hungry, malnourished, and food-insecure people.[70]

There is more methane coming from meat and dairy production than from all transportation sources combined, which is increasing global warming greatly. Think about how much meat and dairy and eggs your family consumes in one week. If we all cut back a little it would make an impact. If we cut back a lot, we would see huge changes. If we cut it out, the world and our health would not even look the same!

My husband loves the sea. We are blessed to live in beautiful San Diego. He went snorkeling recently, came home and said, "It's just not the same. With global warming, the fish population is shrinking and everything looks dead. There are no more starfish and the kelp is dying. It's really sad that this has happened to our Earth and oceans. Our kids will never see what we did because of the destruction we are causing."

Let's not be sad or depressed about this news. Let's change it! Just as your body responds quickly when you stop abusing it, so does our Earth. It's not too late!

CHAPTER 9

THE LESS INGREDIENTS THE BETTER!

Even scientists don't fully understand why an apple a day keeps the doctor away. Our bodies are extremely complex and each food we eat sets off an unfathomable number of reactions in our body. If we eat food that is not natural but processed, and contains ingredients that are known to be unhealthy, what types of reactions are we setting off? In the book *Whole* by Dr. T. Colin Campbell,[71] there is a chart which shows glucose metabolism and other metabolic pathways. It's the most complex chart I've ever seen! Besides confirming my absolute belief in a supreme creator, the master scientist, God, if I want to keep my body working as it's meant to I must eat whole, natural foods to retain or regain my health. As they say, garbage in, garbage out!

The best ingredient list is one with whole food, plant based items, such as an apple, potato, orange, banana, fig, bean, brown rice, strawberry, etc. But when we do purchase something like bread or cereal, try to find one that has the fewest ingredients so you are eating food that's as close to natural as you can. Try to buy 100% whole grains, and not enriched grains or just "whole grains," which is the sneaky term for "not 100% whole grains." Enriched grains are stripped of their goodness with a sprinkle of goodness added back in them. We want all the goodness we can get! Goodness is less addictive than enriched, so eat whole grains for more nutrients, more satisfaction and less desire to overeat. Remember, oils are not whole foods. Oils are processed, nearly pure fat foods. Avoid them for your best health.

CHAPTER 10
IF YOU DON'T KNOW WHAT AN INGREDIENT IS, GOOGLE IT!

IN THIS DAY and age, with a full encyclopedia set and much more in your purse or pocket, take 10 seconds and google an ingredient you don't know. Maybe it's something totally healthy, or maybe it's horrible; now you know. Of course, be careful of your sources and when in doubt, buy real food with real food names.

Read labels with your kids. Don't look for calories; look for ingredients. I love reading labels to my son to try to discourage him from making a bad food choice. I love the scared look he gets on his face when I tell him what he was about to put in his body. It is scary! It's sad that we live in a world where the main stream choices are bad for us foods, and the people turning them down are the "odd" ones, not those feeding themselves poison. Food companies give us what we want, cheap and tasty. Don't fall for it! Choose health!

But everyone else is doing it, eating everything and anything, and they all seem fine and they are happy and they seem healthy and are enjoying life, so why should I change? Here is the reason. This information I'm sharing is true. Avoid future pain and suffering with a whole food, plant based diet.

CHAPTER 11

READ THE LABEL!

You want your food to be full of goodness, not disease causing agents. Whole foods are what we should be eating, not packaged processed foods. So really our foods should not even have labels. I know that we live in a world of processed foods and we don't all eat whole foods 100% of the time, even though that should be our goal. When you do buy something processed, do your best to buy the least damaging foods you can. Stop looking at the protein, carbohydrate, sodium, fat and calorie count and look at the ingredients. That's all you need to know.

On a food label the company lists the ingredients from the most used in the recipe to the least. You don't want the worst foods listed in the top of the list; completely avoid them if you can.

Fat free—remember those days when everything was fat free, and then we found out that our food was filled with sugar instead? So then we went sugar free by filling our food with chemical sweeteners and filling our foods with oils that are "healthy." Wow, that's a whole lot of confusion!

Try to avoid these foods on your labels: Any animal proteins, meat, dairy or eggs. Next, avoid processed soy. Next, avoid chemicals of any type; and finally, avoid processed sugar. Look for whole, organic if you can afford it, ingredients that are grains, fruits and vegetables. If you can't find what you want with the ingredients you want, try making your own, like baked tortilla chips. See the easy recipe for tortilla chips in my recipe section.

You definitely don't want sugar to be one of the first ingredients listed. Sugar feeds cancer. Sugar feeds yeast, leading to overgrowth.

Sugar feeds disease. But don't forget, we learned that animal protein turns on the growth of tumors so avoid animal proteins[72] before you avoid sugar. Remember that sugar is listed under a lot of names. Don't be fooled by how much sugar there really is in a food just because you don't know all the names for sugar.

Common Names for Sugar
According to the U.S. Dept. of Health and Human Services (HHS), added sugars show up on food and drink labels under the following names: Anhydrous dextrose, brown sugar, cane crystals, cane sugar, corn sweetener, corn syrup, corn syrup solids, crystal dextrose, evaporated cane juice, fructose sweetener, fruit juice concentrates, high-fructose corn syrup, honey, liquid fructose, malt syrup, maple syrup, molasses, pancake syrup, raw sugar, sugar, syrup and white sugar. Other types of sugar that you might commonly see on ingredient lists are fructose, lactose and maltose. Fructose is sugar derived from fruit and vegetables; lactose is milk sugar; and maltose is sugar that comes from grain.

Less Common Names for Sugar
The HHS list of sugar names is by no means exhaustive. According to the non-profit Food Label Movement, there are almost 100 different names for sugar and sugar alcohols on ingredient lists. Some of the less apparent sugar names include carbitol, concentrated fruit juice, corn sweetener, diglycerides, disaccharides, evaporated cane juice, erythritol, Florida crystals, fructooligosaccharides, galactose, glucitol, glucoamine, hexitol, inversol, isomalt, maltodextrin, malted barley, malts, mannitol, nectars, pentose, raisin syrup, ribose rice syrup, rice malt, rice syrup solids, sorbitol, sorghum, sucanat, sucanet, xylitol and zylose.[73]

When baking at home, I use 100% pure maple syrup for sweetening things and really, it does not take much. Luckily we recently found that Costco carries 100% pure maple syrup for half the price of the health food stores so buy it there if you want to save a few bucks!

Under no circumstances should you eat fake sugar! Why not, you ask? What is that fake sugar doing to your body? It's not natural, it's processed, and it could have terrible effects on your health. Is it worth eating the unknown? What if you are diabetic? Again, please see Dr. McDougall's lecture, Diabetes, drugs and 100 years of missed opportunities[74], at https://www.drmcdougall.com/health/education/videos/free-electures/diet-drugs-and-diabetes/.

Pick up any packaged food and you'll be shocked if it does not contain some type of oil or even multiple types. As consumers we've been brainwashed to believe that oil is a healthy food; but oil is just fat extracted out of something, and eating pure fat is not healthy. Even plant fat is not good if you eat it in a processed form. Plant fats are great and in the amounts we need, and mixed with the other nutrients we need when we eat a whole food. Cut out the oils.

CHAPTER 12

IT'S CHEAPER TO EAT HEALTHY

Many people mistakenly believe that plant-based eating is more expensive, but it doesn't have to be. What can get expensive quickly is buying lots of "faux" meats and cheeses (real meat and cheese is already costly), packaged and prepared food, and takeout. A diet composed of simple, wholesome ingredients can actually cost less than one that includes meat.[75]

Rice, beans, oats and potatoes are some of the cheapest foods on the planet. They might not satiate your SAD (Sad American Diet) palate at first; but in time and with some seasonings they will, and to a much greater extent than you ever thought possible. Of course, on a whole food, plant based diet you can eat much more than rice, beans, oats and potatoes, but those are a few quickies to get you started. This should also help you see that healthy eating is quite possible, even on a limited budget.

I've learned that when there is a will there is a way, so make up your mind to eat healthy and then figure out a plan to make it work for your family, your schedule and your budget. No excuses! I saved a lot of money when I switched from a veggie diet with a lot of nuts and seeds and oils to a starch based diet. Starches are much cheaper than animal foods, too. Starches really are the cheapest foods out there, the best for your body and mind, and the most satiating. It's sad that carbs have been demonized, all in the name of profits.

Your body is an amazing and beautiful creation that is wonderfully complex and sensitive. Treat your body like the gift it is. You would not buy an expensive sports car and fill it with cheap gas, right? How much more important is it to treat your body right? You want your body to last a healthy 100 years, right? Fuel it for the long haul!

CHAPTER 13

IN THE BEGINNING, THERE WAS FOOD

I LISTENED TO a beautiful lecture by Dr. Scott Stoll. This lecture was from the McDougall Advanced Study Weekend, February 12-14th, 2016 in Santa Rosa California. I purchased and watched a recording of the event online. I love Dr. Stoll's demeanor. He's very excited that he can help his patients to change their life by changing their diet, and I love his big smile and kind encouragement. In his lecture[76] he said, "in the beginning there was food." He showed the loveliest photos of fruits and veggies and grains I think I've ever seen. It really was breathtaking. This food was perfectly healthy and perfectly packaged (inside the skin of the fruit, etc.) with all the nutrients we need. It was glorious and beautiful and lovely and we ate it and were abundantly healthy and satisfied. But then we changed the food and we can't figure out why we are all getting sick. As I've learned in many areas of my life, when I get off track I need to go back to the basics. The basics of good health are starches, fruits and vegetables. Why would we want to go back to the basics? The basics will save our health and to save our planet.

Dr. Stoll said that his patients were coming to his office and they would always say the same thing. "Doctor, I'm falling apart." At first, his only answers were an injections, surgery or pills. He says that not only were they falling apart, but their lives were falling apart as well. They had bad marriages because of their health troubles, they couldn't visit their grandkids because of their pain, and they were in financial ruin because they couldn't work. They really were falling apart. He didn't know what to do.

He said from 1931 to 1999 there were over 900 diet studies done. Most of those diets had an average weight loss of 20 to 24 pounds, but after five years the diets only had a 15% success rate. These diets were fads and hard to stick to, and people would go back to their old habits because they could not stick to a diet that didn't satiate their bodies.

Dr. Stoll found that a plant based diet was the one treatment that really helped his patients, more than anything else he could do for them. He said that eating the right food changes lives. It affects every aspect of life. He started to write prescriptions for patients for a plant based diet. Dr. Stoll says that 63% of the American diet is processed food, 25% is animal food and 12% is plant food; but really half of that plant food is made up of ketchup, fries and juice. Dr. Stoll has found that plant-based food needs to be the cornerstone of your diet. This cornerstone will help the world from the atomic level all the way to the global level. Plant based nutrition helps with anti-aging, it lowers blood pressure, prevents heart disease, cancer, IBS, dementia, plus improves brain function and improves your bones, kidney, liver, etc. You'll feel better every day with a plant-based diet. You will have less sick days, less pain and you will be more active. Your relationships will be better. You will save money on healthcare. Dr. Stoll is enthusiastic about gardening, and I'm really excited about the things I've learned from him through his introduction to the movie *Back to Eden,* about organic gardening made easy. Dr. Stoll says we need to work together in our communities to bring this healthy cornerstone to pass.

Dr. Stoll states that in our nation it's predicted that we will have a 100% increase in diabetes by the year 2030. In developing countries, by 2030 cancer will be the number one killer, overtaking heart disease. And 75% of the cancers will be in developing countries because they are adopting our way of eating.

In his lecture, Dr. Stoll says that 75% of our healthcare costs, which currently are $2.85 trillion, are directly caused by our poor diet. Imagine what we could do with that money—help those in need instead of trying to save ourselves from the poison we eat. Dr. Stoll mentioned that it takes two football fields to feed one person the standard American diet, but it also takes two football fields to feed 14 people a plant based diet. If all 7 billion people on Earth wanted to eat the standard American diet, we would need two Earths to have enough resources, such as land, water and energy to feed everybody. Dr. Stoll commented that it takes 12,000 gallons of water to feed a family of four for a year on a plant-based diet but it also takes 12,000 gallons of water to produce 10 pounds of beef. What you eat today has a profound impact on the globe.

Dr. Stoll recommended five steps to a whole food plant-based healthy food cornerstone diet. 1. Get rid of processed food and dairy. 2. Get rid of animal products. 3. Eat more whole plant foods. 4. Buy organic for "the dirty dozen." 5. Grow your own food.

Some people say that herbicides and pesticides are terrible for you and we should try to avoid them. While it is best to buy organic foods, or even better to grown you own food, Dr. Stoll says that even fruits and veggies that are sprayed with pesticides are better than animal products for our health.

I love the truth of his message; that in the beginning there were grains, fruits and vegetables, and it was glorious and beautiful and healthy and satisfying, and perfectly complete and whole; and it was good and we should keep eating that same way for our optimal health and the health of our family, community, nation and our planet.

CHAPTER 14

PINK SALT FOR EVERYONE

SALT IS NOT the enemy. Sprinkle a bit on your food to add to your enjoyment. The foods that are really high in sodium are processed foods, not whole foods, so adding a bit of salt to your whole foods is fine. Try using a less processed salt like Pink Himalayan salt, or a sea salt that has the minerals your body needs.

Himalayan crystal salt is far superior to traditional iodized salt. Himalayan salt is millions of years old and pure, untouched by many of the toxins and pollutants that pervade other forms of ocean salt.

Known in the Himalayas as "white gold," Himalayan Crystal Salt contains the same 84 natural minerals and elements found in the human body. This form of salt has also been maturing over the past 250 million years under intense tectonic pressure, creating an environment of zero exposure to toxins and impurities.

Himalayan salt's unique cellular structure allows it to store vibrational energy. Its minerals exist in a colloidal form, meaning that they are tiny enough for our cells to easily absorb.

Himalayan Crystal Salt: The Health Benefits
The health benefits of using natural Himalayan Crystal Salt may include:

- *Controlling the water levels within the body, regulating them for proper functioning*
- *Promoting stable pH balance in the cells, including the brain.*
- *Encouraging excellent blood sugar health*
- *Aiding in reducing the common signs of aging*

- *Promoting cellular hydroelectric energy creation*
- *Promoting the increased absorption capacities of food elements within the intestinal tract*
- *Aiding vascular health*
- *Supporting healthy respiratory function*
- *Lowering incidence of sinus problems, and promoting over-all sinus health*
- *Reducing cramps*
- *Increasing bone strength*
- *Naturally promoting healthy sleep pattern*
- *Creating a healthy libido*
- *Circulator support*
- *Promotes kidney and gall bladder health when compared to common chemically-treated salt*[77].

Although I am promoting fresh whole foods, I sometime buy food in a can for convenience. I don't always plan ahead or get it all right all the time. The sodium number listed on packaged food should not be higher than the calorie number. Make sure you buy low sodium items, and rinse them before serving to get some of that extra salt off.

When preparing your food, it's best to salt it to your taste at the table instead of using a lot of salt while cooking. When the salt touches your tongue, you taste it more than when it's buried in your food. Less is more when salting at the table instead of at the stovetop.

Salt is not the evil villain we have heard it is, unless you have specific condition that requires you to avoid it. Salt helps a plant based diet be even more enjoyable.

CHAPTER 15

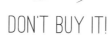

DON'T BUY IT!

DON'T BUY JUNK food, aka processed foods, animal products or oils. Find healthy foods that you love that satisfy your body. When I want a treat, nothing works likes fruit and if it's really serious, I bring out the Medjool dates. Heaven! If you are looking for something a bit more exciting than fruit try my favorite dessert recipe, my No Bake Strawberry Pie in the recipe section at the end of this book. A fruit platter is what we usually have for dessert if anyone is craving something sweet. That might not sound sweet enough for you, but as you choose to eat plant based and your taste adjusts to whole foods, you'll be surprised at how satisfying fruit can be. I remember hearing from others that they ate fruit for dessert, and thinking "I could never do that," but here I am, telling you to try it. If it happened to me, who used to pack chocolate in my suitcase to go on vacation because I couldn't live a day without it, it can happen to you too. It turns out that when you eat a diet your body was built to consume you actually don't crave much. Almost all nights we have no dessert and no-one asks for it. I believe the high glucose content in a starch based diet satisfies our bodies craving for sugar so we don't need to go searching for sweets after we eat.

If we don't want our family or ourselves to eat junk food, we need to stop buying it. I know that sounds obvious, but if you have a craving for a treat and that treat is in the house, if you are like me, you are much more likely to find it and eat it. I'm not willing to drive myself to the store to buy something that will damage my health so it's not as tempting if it's not around. There are lots of whole food, plant based treats as well.[78] Try my no dairy no added sugar Milk Shakes in my recipe section at the end of the book. It's one of my kids' favorites! Yum!

For me, it really does not work to say that I will eat healthy most of the time and "cheat" once in a while, like my family does. Cheating keeps my taste alive for junk, and the more I "cheat" the more I want to. Our Standard American Diet (SAD) is highly addictive. You know, you've tasted it. Like any habit you want to break, it's best to steer clear of the temptation completely. The best way to stop is to stop, if you really want to break the SAD chains.

CHAPTER 16

TROUBLEMAKERS

THREE FOODS, MEAT, dairy and eggs cause heart disease, diabetes, cancer and obesity, just to name a few. Eat them sparingly or not at all. Dr. Colin Campbell of *The China Study* says that you can eat up to 5% of your food from meat and dairy before it starts to cause disease and they literally turned cancer growth on and off by increasing or decreasing the amount of casein (milk protein) the lab rats were fed.[79] I realize that humans are not lab rats; however the test was done in China, with people, and the results were the same. In China, people were not forced or even asked to eat an increased amount of animal protein. The study was tracking what large populations were already doing and seeing the results on their health.[80]

It's too bad that we don't have an immediate reaction to things that are bad for us. It sometimes takes 40+ years for our bodies to no longer be able to fight back against the poisons we feed it. What a true blessing we have in our amazing bodies; we can mistreat them for so long and they still serve us well, for decades for most people!

How about moderation? As we've learned from Dr. Colin Campbell, you can eat 5% of your diet as animal protein before it causes tumor growth.[81] If you know that animal protein is not good for you and you want to have the best health possible, why eat it at all? Do we smoke sparingly if we are trying to quit or drinking sparingly if we are an alcoholic trying to be sober? NO! Likewise, if we are addicted to animal proteins and fat filled food, eating "mostly healthy," with cheating here and there will keep our taste alive for foods that damage and disease our bodies but feed our emotional and physical desires. It's really best to eat 100% healthy. The cool part is that you really won't miss that food once you stop eating it. You will also develop a new appreciation for the delicious taste of food just the way God made it. The other night we were eating a delicious stir fry and I told my husband that it tasted as good as ice cream used to taste to me with no negative side effects. It was true! I could not stop eating it!

Americans die from diseases of affluence like diabetes, heart disease and cancer. Some people argue against a healthy diet by saying that we are all going to die anyway, so let's just live it up! What they night not realize is that this statement can mean means dialysis machines, amputations, a cracked chest for bypass surgery, chemotherapy, radiation, and a slew of prescription drugs that make you feel horrible. Does eating a whole food, plant based diet really prevent these things? YES!

After just going through two and a half years of terrible and chronic back pain (after I broke my back, and then had surgery that still didn't fix my back), plus prior health issues and surgeries, I know that anything is worth relieving future suffering. I'm happy to eat healthy food now so I can have a healthy future. I try to instill this in my children, which is harder to do since they've never really felt much pain or discomfort and grew up on the Standard American Diet. I guess my explanations are working though, because most of them are doing a pretty good job of making good food choices. It warms my heart!

CHAPTER 17

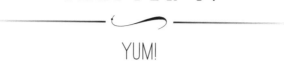

YUM!

WHOLE FOODS ARE actually delicious and flavorful but Americans and many other nations drown their food in gravy, oils, MSG, Ranch dressing, and chemical additives, fry their food, salt it, add corn syrup, etc. Do you know how much sugar you are eating? It's in everything. When I started eating more healthy foods and making food choices based on what would make my body feel vibrant, I stopped topping my food with things like Parmesan cheese. At first my food tasted a bit bland, but in no time at all my taste buds adjusted and the simplest food was delicious. I could taste the natural, delicious flavor of the food. Now, the thought of putting dips and sauces on my food that are not made of natural seasonings and are full of fat and chemicals and animal products makes me cringe. It makes my food taste worse, not better, and turns my healthy food into unhealthy food.

I feel so much better when I eat healthy food. In the past I'd make something like macaroni and cheese for my kids and sneak a spoonful or two or three or five or 10! Then I'd feel guilty for eating the extra calories, and I'd feel sick to my stomach from the butter and milk. Later I'd have a bad taste in my mouth from the dairy and have to chew gum to cover the bad taste. Then I'd weigh myself in the morning and beat myself up over the number I saw and try to live on vegetables the next day. Not a fun way to live!

Natural food really is delicious. Give it a chance. Give it some time. Before you know it, you will love the plain and pure and simple food too with no guilt, no disease and no extra weight on your body. Did you hear that? You can eat as much food as you want and never gain weight by eating starches like grains, beans, potatoes plus fruits and veggies. I spent so much of my life on a limited calorie diet trying to watch my weight that it really is thrilling to eat until I am full and satisfied at every meal.

CHAPTER 18

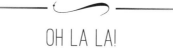

OH LA LA!

In 2011 I invited a friend of mine, (Kelli who you will meet later in this book,) to go to a spa with me. She is a super-fit yoga teacher and model, and I was really excited to go but I was super-nervous about being seen in a bathing suit, especially with her walking next to me. I knew that no matter what I did, I just could not possibly look good next to her. I was in pretty good shape, but I was definitely not comfortable with my body. I had a few extra pounds on my thighs that I really was not fond of. Being an exercise addict and a calorie counting junkie, I didn't know what more I could do to get my body to look as I wanted it to, other than eating "perfectly" 100% of the time. That seemed impossible, and I was not sure I even wanted to live like that; it was so hard to restrict myself all the time and not cave into my food addictions or a pleasure eat. At that time, I was totally confused as to what it even meant to eat perfectly. Back then, I'd probably say to never eat dessert would be perfect, and I thought that animal protein was good for me! As time went on, and I went through breaking my back and all the crazy health issues that followed, my diet got much better and I learned that my previous "perfect" version of eating was not even close to perfect. There was a way that I could really be healthy and never worry about weight again if I ate within certain parameters which were very satisfying and healthy. I went from counting calories to counting health.

When I look back, I was really not eating a diet that could be duplicated with my first version of what I thought "healthy" meant. Most of the time, I was full but unsatisfied. I ate a ton of veggies (literally) but my body wanted carbs! Fuel! Energy! I would allow myself to eat carbohydrates but only once a day, because I thought they were bad for me, causing blood sugar spikes, weight gain and all those bad rumors you hear. So I was eating mostly veggies and fruit, small amounts of grains and lots of nuts, what I thought were healthy oils, and avocados. I later read *The Starch Solution*,[82] and Dr. McDougall helped me to understand that I needed more starch and less fat. I changed my diet to his diet plan and I have never felt better. My plate is now full of fruits and veggies and starches like grains, potatoes, beans, brown rice, and corn. I never count calories, I'm never hungry, and I have stopped weighing myself every day. What a blessing! This is the diet I will eat for the rest of my life. It's very low fat and super heart-healthy. I don't just want to look good on the outside, I want to be healthy on the inside too, and this diet is helping me to accomplish both.

Dr. Esselstyn says that you are heart attack proof when your cholesterol is 150 or less,[83] and that heart disease is a toothless paper tiger.[84] How awesome it is to be heart attack proof! The biggest killer in America can be totally avoided!

So why don't doctors tell you this? There are several reasons. For one, it's hard to make a living telling patients to eat healthy food when they could be telling patients they need expensive medication and a $20,000 stent or five instead! Also, medical doctors for the most part don't learn preventative medicine. They learn to treat health issues with pharmaceuticals and surgery. The next issue is that people in general really don't want to take care of their bodies. They want the easy way out. They want a pill to cover their bad habits. The problem is that the pills don't make them feel true, vibrant health; they just cover some of the symptoms while creating new symptoms to deal with. It's a big tradeoff. These are not great choices, but most people cooperate and follow the doctor's orders. Instead, choose health. It's the cheapest, easiest and best answer for a long, healthy life. A healthy life translates into a happy life, because you feel wonderful and free and you don't make decisions based on your health. I remember the miserable days of deciding what I could and could not due based on my back pain. What a terrible and frustrating way to live!

My diet is based on Dr. McDougall's plan, *The Starch Solution*, which also matches up with Dr. Esselstyn's plan to prevent and reverse heart disease, and also Dr. Colin Campbell's plan to stop cancer from starting. It also aligns with my church's diet recommendations that I never seemed to be able to follow in the past. I could never convince most friends or my children to eat my veggie diet because it was hard and expensive and unsatisfying. A whole food, plant based diet is so much better! I really believe in it and it's really simple, cheap, easy and satisfying. I feel so blessed to have found this truth.

When I was eating the SAD Diet (Standard American Diet) also known as the Toxic American Diet, food tasted amazing but I did not feel amazing. I had lots of tummy aches, lots of intestinal upset, breakouts, and I definitely did not like how my body looked. I finally ended up cutting out gluten and my intestines were happy again. I don't think that most people need to cut out gluten but I somehow developed a bad reaction to it during my fourth pregnancy and it stayed with me. There is nothing at all wrong with eating wheat. The findings in the book *Grain Brain and Wheat Belly*, says Dr. McDougall,[85] are based on the findings from tests done with people who have Celiac Disease, so please don't think you need to cut out gluten. It is best to buy non-GMO, organic and pesticide free for all your grains, if you can.

Later in my diet experimentation, I cut out dairy and my tummy felt so much better! It's amazing that it took years of not feeling well and not looking how I wanted to look before I was willing to make some changes. Now I'm so glad I did! It also took me looking for information about healthy eating, because I really didn't know what true healthy eating was and I hadn't spent the time to find out. I just stayed on 25 years of miserable diets before getting out of the passenger seat and taking the wheel.

The food I make now is simple, delicious and nutritious, and I choose it because it will improve my health, and my family's health. If you are not feeling great, start a journal of what you eat and drink, the number of hours you sleep and the stress in your life. Journal everything you put in your mouth for two weeks and also write down any reactions that happen after you eat that particular food. Also write down any reactions after particular thoughts or feeling or interactions that effect you negatively. If you find a food that bothers you, stop eating it! If you find a thought, feeling, person, situation that is not for your best good, change it! Note the changes in your health and don't look back. Some people can't eat foods that one would consider healthy. That's okay! Listen to your body and eat healthy foods that make you feel great. Some people have food allergies that clear up once they are on a whole food, plant based diet or once they clear out the junk in their minds too.

But what if you are thin and don't feel bad when you eat animal products? You may be one of those blessed with a quick metabolism, or no desire for emotional eating, and no allergies; but eating meat, dairy, eggs, oils and still feeling good does not mean that you are not damaging your body internally, and that is even worse. Six hundred thousand Americans drop dead every year from heart disease alone, not to mention all the other diseases and cancers that abound. There is one recipe for health that works for everyone. You don't need to be a certain blood type. No matter who you are, a whole food, plant based diet will give you the best chance at health and fitness for your whole life. Choose health!

CHAPTER 19

WHAT IS HEALTH FOOD?

WITH SO MANY diets out there, it's almost impossible to know what we really should be eating. I think we can all agree that broccoli and all greens are healthy but beyond that there are inconsistencies. Some diets don't even let you eat fruit. Do other diets besides a whole food, plant based diet work for losing weight? Absolutely! But the goal is not just weight loss, although you will absolutely have that with a whole food, plant based diet. The goal is health, vitality and no disease! The best way to eat to have the health you want, the body you want, and the energy you want is to eat a whole food, plant based diet. How can you know that this is the best diet? Because it prevents and reverses disease and keeps you feeling full and satisfied unlike any other diet. Your body will stay healthy, or heal itself if needed, but only with the right fuel.

Try this healthy prescription: For breakfast, have oatmeal with berries on top or pancakes made from whole grains—see my recipe section for my favorite pancakes. For a snack, grab fruits and veggies. For lunch, have a big salad with beans and sprouts or lentils and if heart disease is not a risk factor for you (and your cholesterol is under 150) put a small sprinkle of nuts or avocado on top. For a dressing use vinegar and lemon or try my dressing recipe in the recipe section. Have some grapes or veggies with oil-free hummus for an afternoon snack. For dinner, have some brown rice with grilled or steamed veggies and a whole food sauce or spaghetti or potato and vegetable soup. The options are really endless, delicious, and nutritious. This is the kind of fuel your body needs to perform as it was meant to.

Why is it so hard to know what healthy food is? Lots of people have lots of opinions! What are those opinions based on? And are they trying to sell you something? My favorite books that teach a whole food, plant based diet and also prove how this way of life will prevent and reverse disease and make you slim and vibrant and healthy are: *The China Study* by Dr. T. Colin Campbell,[86] which is the most in-depth study ever done on the relationship between eating animal products and disease; *Prevent and Reverse Heart Disease* by Dr. Esselstyn[87] proves that you can reverse and prevent heart disease by eating a whole food, plant based diet; and *The Starch Solution* by Dr. John McDougall[88] really helps you to understand the lies we've been taught, and what the truth really is about why your body was made to run on starches. Dr. McDougall has been promoting this diet for 40 years! His website is the biggest one stop shop for information I've found, and it's all FREE! Check out www.Dr.McDougall.com.[89] He currently has free weekly webinars on all the hottest health topics, not to mention classes, certifications, recipes and even vacations that only serve a whole food, plant based diet. How great is that?

There really is no secret about what the best diet is if you will take the time to do some study and look at the science from unbiased sources. Make sure the studies you are reading are not funded by the meat, dairy or egg industry.

CHAPTER 20

SUSTAINABILITY

HERE IS THE truth. We are eating 70 billion animals per year. That is unfathomable! We can't keep eating animals at this rate for so many reasons beyond just our health. First, it takes so many resources to feeds all those animals. We are using up plant food we could be using to feed the world's poor, but instead we are fattening up animals for the slaughter because that's what we want to eat. People are literally dying of starvation because the cost of grains has gone above their ability to pay for them, due to the supply and demand of our selfish desires to eat the richest food all day, every day. Yes, "The Man in The Mirror[90]" song just popped into my head. It is time to make a change. Thank you, Michael!

Guess what produces more greenhouse gases that all the transportation vehicles combined? Methane from animals! Do we not know? Do we not care? I didn't know about this before I started researching. How can we not know this? When will we start think about our health, having enough food for all, kindness to animals, and the health of our planet?

Production of animals for consumption takes a lot of water too. Right now, we are in a drought in California (where I live) so why not eat more plant food and save the water that would be used to produce animals? From watching the movie *Cowspiracy*,[91] I learned that it takes 660 gallons of water to produce one hamburger. So take a longer shower and cut the meat you eat and you will still be saving a lot of water.

Part of the problem is that we don't know how to make dinner without meat. What would we make? Would our family complain? Feel deprived? Since we've been lead to believe that we NEED animal products to be healthy, do we believe that it is a lie, or do we think that we will harm our family's health by not feeding them animal products? Do we feel too busy to take the time to do the research? If you feel that you don't have enough time to investigate this, think a little more about the importance of this topic. Your health and the health of generations to come are counting on you. This topic is worthy of your study. I guess I am preaching to the choir since you are reading this book. Good for you! Hopefully my years of research, condensed into this book, will save you some time, answer your questions, and give you the motivation that you need to make changes.

What about the way we treat other living creatures? While views differ about the degree of comfort and freedom that farm animals deserve, most people can agree on a minimum standard of cleanliness and space, and that animals should not suffer needlessly. Yet the reality is that the basic structure of industrial farms is at odds with the overall well-being of the animals they raise.

Industrial farms push for the maximum production from the animals regardless of the stress this places them under and the resultant shortening of their lifespan. Confining as many animals indoors as possible might maximize efficiency and profits, but it also exposes the animals to high levels of toxins from decomposing manure and can create ideal conditions for diseases to spread. Feeding animals an unnatural diet rather than letting them graze and forage on open land simply adds to their health problems. To counteract these unhealthy conditions, factory farmed animals are given constant low doses of antibiotics[92] that are contributing to the development of antibiotic-resistant bacteria. Factory farmed animals are also routinely treated with pesticides[93] and other unhealthy additives,[94] and can be given hormones[95] solely to increase productivity.[96]

I really didn't know these truths until I started researching health. Now I know. Knowledge is power. Let's be the change!

CHAPTER 21

VITAMINS AND SUPPLEMENTS

VITAMINS AND SUPPLEMENTS turn our focus to the wrong issue. Have you ever met anyone with a vitamin deficiency disease? Not in today's world of over-nutrition. It's not a vitamin or mineral or supplement that will fix the major health issues of today, it's eating right.

If there is one thing I've learned in my study of health, it's that our bodies are amazingly complex. I knew that before I started studying health, but the deeper I delve into trying to understand, I realize how little I know. The exciting part is you really don't need to understand health. It's important to learn a few keys facts, such as animal protein, oils, processed foods and food additives cause disease and destroy our Earth. When you run one medical test, it's really hard to prove that while one supplement, for example, might have helped you in a certain way, it didn't harm you in another. Your body is one constant complex chain of chemical reactions. Maybe a calcium tablet increased your calcium, but what else did it do? I've seen many studies[97] showing the damage that Americans do to themselves by taking vitamins and supplements. Of course, prescription drugs do much worse damage, but the point I want to make is please don't take a vitamin or supplement just to take it. If you have a vitamin or mineral issue with your body, first make sure that you are eating right. If you still have problems with your body, go to see a doctor who specializes in herbal remedies, pay for a high quality product and use it if it's helping you. I believe in muscle testing. A muscle test allows your body to tell you what it needs. Don't go to the grocery store and buy vitamins, minerals, fish oil, vitamin D and calcium just because you heard it's good for you. You will most likely be doing more harm than good and/or wasting a lot of money.

Eating the Western diet causes serious common chronic diseases. In an effort to heal, the body responds with repair processes that include inflammation. One of the responses to this inflammation is the lowering of the serum 25-hydroxyvitamin D in the blood. Thus, low vitamin D in the blood is a result of being ill, not the cause of sickness. This is the main the reason studies using vitamin D supplements have consistently shown no benefits to patients with common chronic diseases. The metabolic imbalances created by administrating this unnatural substance may actually be responsible for the increase in falls, fractures, and other damage. (Vitamin D is a hormone synthesized with the help of sunlight; it is not intended for oral intake or injection.)

Studies show, in addition to the healing processes, that even our basic food choices lead to inflammation. Consuming meat and other animal foods increase inflammation while grains and vegetables decrease inflammation. Thus, low vitamin D levels do not cause obesity, heart disease, diabetes, multiple sclerosis, and cancer, but rather result from the illnesses (and the very foods that caused these chronic conditions).[98]

The epidemic of obesity has added to the epidemic of vitamin D deficiency. Because vitamin D is fat soluble, excess body fat will pull vitamin D out of circulation, thus contributing to lower levels.

We've all heard that the soil is depleted of vitamins and minerals, which is why we need supplements even if we are eating our fruits and veggies. First off, fruits and veggies make their own vitamins; they don't come from the soil, so we don't have that issue. Second, although some soils have been found to lack some minerals, especially in Africa, as long as we are eating fruits and veggies that were grown in more than a 25-mile radius of where we live, we are eating food that is grown in a mix of different soils and are getting the minerals we need.

Nearly forty percent of the US population takes supplements, with many people spending hundreds of dollars a month. Based on what objective evidence? How many friends and relatives do you know who have suffered from illnesses caused by a vitamin deficiency, such as scurvy from vitamin C deficiency, beriberi from insufficient vitamin B1, or pellagra from a lack of niacin?

How about protein or essential fatty acid deficiencies? The truth is none. Now, turn your vision 180 degrees. I'll ask you the opposite question.

How many of your friends and relatives have diseases caused by nutritional excesses—from consuming too much cholesterol, fat, sodium, protein and/or far too many calories? The answer is most of them. Health problems from excesses cannot be corrected with treatments useful for deficiencies. Have you ever known a person who has lost 100 pounds by taking supplements or cured their arthritis, hypertension, colitis, or type 2 diabetes through vitamin and mineral therapies? I bet you haven't and neither have I.

Whether you are scientifically minded and believe in the perfection created by 400 million years of evolution, or devoutly religious and believe in the perfection of a Divine Creator, or both, you must believe that the world we live in is inherently correct. The trillions of interactions that occur between flora, fauna and Mother Earth are purposeful and harmonious. You have also observed that man's interference with Nature's mysterious workings usually results in unintended catastrophes. Failure to follow the natural starch-based diet for humans is the reason more than a billion people are overweight and sick today. Trying to fix modern day health problems with supplements adds to the injury at great financial costs. (Sales of dietary supplements to US consumers were $25.2 billion in 2008.) Scientific facts and reasoning call for the blind and misguided faith in supplements to stop.

Randomized Controlled Trials Prove Supplements Are Dangerous

More Cancer
The Alpha Tocopherol, Beta Carotene Cancer Prevention Study Group. *A total of 29,133 male smokers were assigned to one of four regimens: alpha tocopherol (vitamin E) alone, beta-carotene alone, both alpha tocopherol and beta carotene, or a placebo.*

Findings: 18 percent more lung cancer and 8 percent more deaths in those taking the preparations with beta-carotene.

The Beta Carotene and Retinol Efficacy Trial. *A total of 18,314 smokers, former smokers, and workers exposed to asbestos were assigned to take beta carotene and retinol (vitamin A) or a placebo.*

Findings: 17 percent more deaths, 46 percent more lung cancer, and 26 percent more cardiovascular disease for those taking the supplement.

The Selenium and Vitamin E Cancer Prevention Trial (SELECT). *A total of 35,533 men were assigned to one of four groups: selenium, vitamin E, selenium plus vitamin E, or a placebo.*

Findings:
Thirteen percent more prostate cancer in the vitamin E groups. No prevention of prostate cancer by any supplement intervention.

More Heart Disease

MRC/BHF Heart Protection Study. *A total of 20,536 adults with coronary disease, other occlusive arterial disease, or diabetes were allocated to receive antioxidant vitamin supplementation (vitamin E, vitamin C, and beta-carotene daily) or a placebo.*

Findings: Increased vitamin concentrations in the subjects' blood, but no reductions in vascular disease, cancer, or death.

Alpha Tocopherol Beta Carotene Cancer Prevention Study. *A total of 1862 male smokers who had had a previous myocardial infarction were assigned to dietary supplements of alpha tocopherol, beta-carotene, both, or a placebo.*

Findings: There were 75% more deaths from fatal coronary artery disease in the beta carotene groups and a slight increase in the alpha tocopherol groups.

The HOPE-TOO trial. *A total of 9541 patients were assigned to vitamin E or a placebo.*

Findings: No difference in cancer or cardiovascular deaths. Patients in the vitamin E group had a higher risk of heart failure.

Folate After Coronary Intervention Trial. *A total of 636 patients with heart artery stents were assigned to receive folic acid, vitamin B6, and vitamin B12 or placebo.*

Findings: Greater restenosis (artery closure) and repeat heart surgery for those taking the supplement with folic acid.

The NORVIT Trial. *A total of 3749 men and women who had had an acute myocardial infarction within seven days were assigned to be in one of five* *groups taking folic acid, vitamin B12 and vitamin B6; folic acid and vitamin B12; vitamin B6; or placebo.*

Findings: Homocysteine decreased by 27 percent, but the risk of heart attack, stroke, and cancer was increased by 20 to 30 percent in the groups with the folic acid supplement.

Women's Antioxidant and Folic Acid Cardiovascular Study *A group of 5442 women with either a history of cardiovascular disease, or three or more coronary risk factors were assigned to receive either folic acid, vitamin B6 and vitamin B12, or a placebo.*

Findings: Homocysteine decreased by 19 percent, but the risk of heart attacks, strokes, heart surgery, and death was not reduced.

More Kidney Damage in Diabetics
The Diabetic Intervention with Vitamins to Improve Nephropathy Trial. *A total of 238 participants who had type 1 or type 2 diabetes and a clinical diagnosis of diabetic nephropathy (kidney disease) were assigned to take folic acid, vitamin B6 and vitamin B12, or a placebo.*

Findings: The groups taking vitamins had worse kidney function and twice as many vascular events.

More Fractures in Elderly
High Dose Oral Vitamin D Trial. *A total of 2256 community-dwelling women, aged 70 years or older, were assigned to receive 500,000 IU of Vitamin D (cholecalciferol) or a placebo.*

Findings: Women taking the vitamin D had more falls and fractures.

More Severe Respiratory Infections
A Randomized Trial on Vitamin E and Infections. *A total of 652 non-institutionalized elderly were assigned to take a multivitamin with minerals, 200 mg of vitamin E, both, or a placebo.*

Findings: No change in the frequency of respiratory infections, but the severity was worse in those taking vitamin E[99].

If you are eating a plant based diet and are still having health challenges, I've learned that our emotions have a lot to do with our health. You could do a muscle test with your chiropractor that says you are in need of an herb to help your adrenal glands for example, but what is causing the adrenal stress? Would it be better to look at the cause and see if you could fix the root of the issue? Yes!

CHAPTER 22

FLU SHOTS AND MORE

SHOTS AND VACCINES are a hot topic for sure, and if you feel like getting into a heated debate with almost anyone, just bring this topic up. So it's with great care that I share my thoughts here with you.

Let's start with the flu shot. Can anyone deny that we are told we need a flu shot? I mean seriously, it's on the "please hold" music at the drug store, it's required for some jobs, it's on posters and banners at the grocery store and in your doctor's office; it's everywhere. You can even get a discount on your groceries at some stores if you get your flu shot. So, the question is, is it really effective and do the drug companies really care that much that we don't get the flu this season, or is it just a money maker with marginal results, if any?

Dr. McDougall posted the graph[100] below in his November 2015 newsletter which shows case studies of the effectiveness of the flu shot. Here are the results, and reasons why I don't get flu shots.

Summary Reports Show the Scarcity of Benefits:[101]
2010 Cochrane Review found no benefits from vaccinating the **elderly**.
2012 Cochrane Review showed little benefit for **children**: "No benefits for those two years or younger. Twenty-eight children over the age of six needed to be vaccinated to prevent one case of influenza. **2012 Lancet Infectious Disease Review** showed little benefit **in adults**: " evidence for consistent high-level protection was elusive for the present generation of vaccines, especially in individuals at risk of medical complications or those aged 65 years or older."

> **2013 Cochrane Review** found no benefits for **healthcare workers** or for preventing influenza in **elderly residents** in long-term care facilities.
>
> **2014 European Review** found that the 2012-2013 influenza vaccine had low to moderate effectiveness, and recommended that seasonal influenza vaccines be improved to achieve acceptable protection levels.
>
> **2014 Cochrane Review** found the preventive effect for **healthy adults** was small: " at least 40 people would need vaccination to avoid one influenza-like illness...no effect on working days lost or hospitalization seen benefits for **pregnant women** were uncertain or at least very limited."

Regarding standard vaccines, this is a topic I will leave for each parent to decide for their children. I highly recommend you read books on the risks verses the benefits of each immunization and then decide how to proceed. It's a huge decision, and one that should not be taken lightly or left unconsidered. Don't get vaccines for your kids because everyone else is doing it and your doctor says you should. Spend some time and decide wisely. If you are religious, this is a decision I would pray over. It's a big decision! A book I read and recommend on vaccines is The Vaccine Book by Robert Sears[102], who calls himself a pro-information doctor. He gives great information to help you make an informed choice on each vaccine. He also has a website at www.thevaccinebook.com[103] or on Facebook at www.facebook.com/dr-bob-sears.[104]

CHAPTER 23

WATER FIRST

DRINK A GLASS of water before anything else every morning. The health benefits are endless!

Why do We Need to Drink Water in the Morning?[105]

- *About 70% of the human body content is water, and so water plays an important role in the proper functioning of your body.*
- *The human brain contains about 85% water.*
- *Your muscles are 75% water.*
- *Bones also contain about 25% water.*
- *Your blood consists of 82% water.*

It is also helpful to consume foods that contain lots of water; for example, soups (broth-based), vegetables and fruits.

What Are the Benefit of Drinking Water in the Morning?

It is a long known secret that drinking water as soon as you get up, i.e. before eating anything, is a good way to purify your internal system. One of the most important results of undergoing this treatment is colon cleansing, which enables better absorption of the nutrients from various foods. When there is production of haematopoiesis, better known as "new blood," you will have immense body restorative effects and you can even be cured of existing ailments. Drinking water the first thing in the morning has the following benefits:

- **Make your skin glow.** *Water is known to purge toxins from your blood, and as a result you get glowing skin.*
- **Renew cells.** *Drinking water first thing in the morning increases the rate at which new muscle and blood cells are produced.*

- ***Balance the lymph system.*** *When you drink water first thing in the morning on a daily basis, you help balance your body's lymph system. Your lymph glands and lymph system fight infections, helping you to perform your daily activities. They also balance the fluids in your body.*
- ***Lose weight.*** *When you consume about 16 ounces of water (chilled), you will boost your body's metabolism by about 24%, thus helping you to lose those extra pounds.*
- ***Purify the colon.*** *When you drink water after you have woken up and before eating anything, you are purifying your colon thereby making nutrients absorption easy.*

Speaking of what to drink, drink water. Remember we are going for whole foods, not parts of the food like the juice of a fruit or veggie. If you are in the mood for an orange or an apple, eat one. Don't sacrifice the fiber or other nutrients you are throwing away or the beneficial metabolic processes whole foods cause in your body. Instead of juice, put a few slices of lemons or limes or cucumber or berries in your water. Juice is too high in calories and sugar too. I say "don't worry about calories," but that is when you are eating whole plant based foods, not foods that are extracted, concentrated or processed.

CHAPTER 24

THE TRUTH ABOUT AMERICANS' HEALTH

IT'S SAD THAT our beliefs about food have become so warped due to our belief in what the media and advertising tell us, and what's popular. Think about the beliefs you have about food. Where did they come from? Have you ever done any research on the science behind your food beliefs? I used to argue about my food facts and I really didn't have any backing for them besides maybe my scale registered better numbers with some diets, but what about my heart? How was that doing? Sadly, I didn't know or care then, but now I know better. Dr. Scott Stoll was a speaker at the McDougall Advanced Study Weekend, February 12-14, 2016 which I watched online. Dr. Stoll found that the best medicine for his patients was plant based nutrition, not surgery, injections or medication. He's now sharing his message with other healthcare providers to help us feel better at www.Plantricianproject.com. Here are some alarming facts and projections[106] that need to change, and the change starts with us.

Evidence that our dietary guidelines and "disease" management system are failing us.

- *It's estimated that a minimum of 80% of all healthcare dollars are spent on the treatment of conditions that are preventable.*
- *70% of Americans are overweight or obese.*
- *Nearly one-half of the American population will be obese by 2030, according to a 2012 study published in the American Journal of Preventive Medicine.*

- *Childhood obesity has tripled in the last 30 years: One out of three American children is overweight or obese.*
- *37% of our children who are not considered overweight have one or more cardiovascular risk factors.*
- *According to Medicare: Health care expenditures in the United States were nearly $2.6 trillion in 2010, an average of $8,402 per person.*
- *70 million Americans have hypertension, with an elevated risk for stroke and heart attack.*
- *The "War on Cancer" waged by President Nixon began over 40 years ago; yet trends indicate that cancer is expected to become the leading cause of death in the U.S. by 2030, according to an ASCO report.*
- *100,000,000 Americans have diabetes or pre-diabetes, with an increased risk of amputation, heart disease, blindness, and limb loss.*
- *Rates of type 2 diabetes increased by 22% among U.S. adults from 1999 to 2008.*
- *Current trends suggest that one in three children born after 2000 will receive a type 2 diabetes diagnosis (for Hispanic children it is 1 in 2).*
- *Many experts project that type 2 diabetes will be a future global epidemic, with diagnosis projections as high as one in three individuals from industrialized nations that have adopted the standard American diet (SAD).*
- *The share of the economy devoted to health care has increased from 7.2% in 1970 to 17.9% in 2009 and 2010, and is now at 18% of GDP.*
- *The U.S. spends substantially more on health care than other developed countries. As of 2009, health spending in the U.S. was about 90% higher than in many other industrialized countries, yet it ranks near the bottom in health outcomes.*
- *90% of the U.S. senior population consumes prescription drugs; with costs doubling in the last 30 years; complications associated with prescription drugs are the #4 cause of death with 45-50 million adverse events annually.*

- We're experiencing prolonged morbidity, with life expectancy now surpassing 78 years, but with more degenerative disease; this is an alarming combination for U.S. healthcare costs.

The toxic SAD is:

- 63% refined and processed foods—empty calories with no health benefit.
- 25% animal based products: meat, dairy and eggs; disease building blocks laden with fat and dietary cholesterol.
- 12% plant based foods, with 6% of this being from french fries, leaving a paltry 6% of daily caloric intake coming from plant based foods (this number also includes things like fruit juice and ketchup).
- We're consuming an average of 185 pounds of added sugar and sweeteners each year.
- We're consuming an average of 3,400 milligrams of salt a day, more than double the recommended amount (triple the amount recommended by many experts), with the majority derived from processed food.

CHAPTER 25

THE CHINA STUDY

The China Study is a book first published in the United States in January 2005 and had sold over one million copies as of October 2013, making it one of America's best-selling books about nutrition.

The China Study examines the relationship between the consumption of animal products (including dairy) and chronic illnesses such as coronary artery disease, diabetes, breast cancer, prostate cancer and bowel cancer. The authors conclude that people who eat a whole food, plant based/vegan diet, avoiding all animal products including beef, pork, poultry, fish, eggs, cheese and milk, and reducing their intake of processed foods and refined carbohydrates, will escape, reduce or reverse the development of numerous diseases. They write that "eating foods that contain any cholesterol above 0 mg is unhealthy."

The book recommends sunshine exposure or dietary supplements to maintain adequate levels of vitamin D, and supplements of vitamin B12 in the case of complete avoidance of animal products. It criticizes low carbohydrate diets, such as the Atkins diet, which includes restrictions on the percentage of calories derived from carbohydrates. The authors are critical of reductionist approaches to the study of nutrition, whereby certain nutrients are blamed for disease, as opposed to studying patterns of nutrition and the interactions between nutrients.

The book is loosely based on *The China-Cornell-Oxford Project*, a 20-year study–described by *The New York Times* as "the Grand Prix of epidemiology"–conducted by the Chinese Academy of Preventive Medicine, Cornell University and the University of Oxford. T. Colin Campbell was one of the study's directors. The study looked at mortality rates from cancer and other chronic diseases from 1973–75 in 65 counties in China; the data was correlated with 1983–84 dietary surveys and blood work from 100 people in each county. The research was conducted in those counties because they had genetically similar populations that tended, over generations, to live and eat in the same way in the same place. The study concluded that counties with a high consumption of animal based foods in 1983–84 were more likely to have had higher death rates from "Western" diseases as of 1973–75, while the opposite was true for counties that ate more plant foods.[107]

Animal products cause tumor growth and are also full of cholesterol that damages the endothelial lining of your arteries. Half a million people in the United States die each year from heart disease. We are killing ourselves with our forks and knives! Dr. Colin Campbell has proved, over and over again, through his lab tests and live tests that the casein in milk causes tumor growth and can be turned on and off like a light switch with the increasing and decreasing of animal protein consumption. If you don't want heart disease or cancer, stay away from animal products. We've been brainwashed by meat and dairy companies to believe that we need meat and dairy for protein and calcium, but we really don't. We can get plenty of protein and calcium from a whole food, plant based diet. Americans actually eat way too much protein, which causes other health issues. Does dairy have calcium? Yes. But it's also acidic and packed with sugar, so in order for our body to try to remain at a happy and healthy pH balance, our body leaches calcium out of our bones to alkalize itself; so when we pee, we are peeing our bones into the toilet! This is why Americans consume the most dairy products of any country in the world yet have the highest rates of osteoporosis in the world.

Dr. T. Colin Campbell, co-author of *The China Study* says that the casein in milk is the most carcinogenic food ever discovered. It's incredibly amazing and scary to me that big business does not care and is happy to cart in truckloads of milk to innocent young children and tell them it's good for them. Nothing could be further from the truth.

CHAPTER 26

VEGGIE TRAYS ON THE TABLE

My husband has been having fun recently by listening to a comedian who likes to talk about bacon and teases about veggies trays at parties, but in your home there should always be a veggie tray out at snack time, and add some fruit too. I love it when my kids are watching TV and I walk into the living room with a huge veggie or fruit tray, or both, and set it down without saying a word; I walk away and watch as they surround and devour the veggies and fruit. Success! My kids didn't always eat like this. I used to put out bowls of Fish Crackers® and then give them Lunchables®. Sorry kids, I didn't know any better. I mean, I knew that something healthier would be better but they are so cheap and easy! I didn't realize I could actually be giving my kids diseases by feeding them animal products coupled with processed foods laden with chemicals and preservatives and artificial flavor and MSG (monosodium glutamate, which actually kills brain cells while you eat it—seriously!) and dyes.

Another key to getting kids to eat veggies is a good dip. Check out my recipe section for my cashew ranch dressing and my hummus recipes. Yum! Start chopping those veggies and enjoy! If you want some super cute veggie tray ideas to make your veggies even more enticing, check out the vegetable tray photos on Pinterest.[108] So fun!

CHAPTER 27

WHAT TO EAT

WHAT DO YOU eat in a whole food, plant based diet? Fruits, veggies, grains, beans, legumes, corn, potatoes and sweet potatoes. You can add nuts and seeds and avocado if your cholesterol is under 150 and you don't want to lose weight. Can you actually make tasty recipes with those few ingredients? Yes! What about protein? Everything I just mentioned is full of protein and has plenty for your daily needs, even if you are an athlete! You don't need extra fat either. Don't believe the healthy oil myths. You get all the healthy fat you need from your plant based food. Doctors Esselstyn, Campbell and McDougall recommend that you season food with herbs and spices, and they all allow for the use of salt and sugar in small amounts. The recommended "sugar" in the *Prevent and Reverse Heart Disease*[109] is 100% maple syrup, and it's delicious in recipes. I use it for all my sweetening.

One of my favorite things about this diet is the simplicity. It's not hard at all to know what to eat. It is important to have some food on hand so that if you are starving you can quickly pull something already made out of the fridge or pop a potato in the microwave.

It's amazing how quickly your body and tastes buds adjust to this diet. I used to eat so much meat. I didn't even think I could skip my breakfast meat let alone my lunch or dinner meat. Now, the thought of meat and the smell of meat really turns my stomach. A friend took me to lunch today at a nice restaurant and I think there was meat on every plate but mine, and the smell was really getting to me. Odd that a few years ago that smell made my mouth water and now I'm repulsed. The same goes for food toppings like sour cream and desserts. They are so rich, I could not eat it if I wanted to. My body is so happy being fed the fuel it was made to run on. I want anything except plant based food now and that feels great!

I do love cooking and I do love my food! Mexican food is probably my favorite. I love rice, beans, salsa, tomatoes, cilantro, corn tortillas and jalapenos. Yum! I also love baking the corn tortilla shells in the oven for chips or tostadas.

At the end of the book I have some of my favorite recipe creations. Try them out and see what you think. I hope you love them too!

For more tips on what not to eat and why, check out Dr. Esselstyn's frequently asked questions and scroll down to see his more commonly asked questions at http://www.dresselstyn.com/site/faq/.[110]

CHAPTER 28

ANTIBIOTICS

IN THE BOOK Disease-Proof Your Child[111] by Dr. Joel Fuhrman M.D., I've been reading about the overuse of antibiotics and the price we pay for it. In my own family, I must admit that our first pediatrician was anti-antibiotics and I used to get so frustrated with her because I'd bring my sick kids to her and she'd say just let them rest and drink plenty of fluids and they will be fine. Maybe give them some pain killer or fever reducer if necessary. I spent my time and money for that answer?!? After learning what I have about the dangerous and even long term side effects of antibiotic use, I am now grateful to that pediatrician for refusing to give me something for my kids. Most doctors are not as concerned with patient health and are more concerned with pleasing the patient/parent and will happily write a prescription for a 10 day dose of amoxicillin or the like. In the last 10 years the antibiotic prescription rate has gone up 50% in the US. I can just picture these worn out moms bringing their kids to the doctor and they better leave with a prescription! I can also picture what these kids are eating on the way to the doctor's office. Probably some type of processed food or animal product which keeps their bodies from being able to fight these germs in the first place. So the doctor writes a prescription for the child's cold, flu, ear infection, sore or strep throat which are mostly all viral illness, to be fought with an antibiotic made to kill bacteria. Some think that colored mucus means you need an antibiotic but virus turns your mucus colors too so don't jump the gun on the "need" for antibiotics due to that. Let's not forget that the misuse of antibiotics is a multi-billion dollar industry per year in the U.S. which is probably why we don't hear too much complaining from the industry about this mis-use.

What happens to the kids on these antibiotics? "Antibiotic can cause diarrhea, digestive disturbances, yeast overgrowth, bone marrow suppression, seizures, kidney damage, colitis, and life-threatening allergic reactions. The unnecessary over-prescription of antibiotics during past decades has been blamed for the recent emergence of antibiotic-resistant strains of deadly bacteria. Besides these potential risks, in every person who takes an antibiotic, the drug kills a broad assortment of helpful bacteria that live in our digestive tract and aid digestion. It kills the "bad" bacteria, such as those that can complicate an infection, but it also kills these helpful "good" bacteria lining your digestive tract that have properties that protect from future illness.[112]"

When you eat plant based foods you promote the healthy bacteria in your body which crowds out the bad bacteria. When you take antibiotics, you kill these good bacteria. When these good bacteria are killed, your body is more susceptible to disease causing microbes and yeast to grow out of control.[113]

100,000+ people per year die from antibiotic-resistant infections. Many of these could have been easily treated in the past but are now resistant infections from our overuse of antibiotics.

In a double blind study with children with ear infections treated with a placebo verses amoxicillin, the symptoms resolved in 8 days in the treatment group and 9 days with the placebo group. Is it worth risking the health of yourself or your children to recover one day faster?[114]

"The vicious cycle of poor nutrition and the overuse of antibiotics work to place a tremendous disease burden on the future health of our children.[115]"

"The use of antibiotics in early childhood is also a contributor to the increasing incidence of allergies, asthma hay fever and eczema to those receiving multiple antibiotic prescriptions early in childhood.[116]"

Research is now also linking the use of antibiotics to Chron's disease. You are also more likely to be diagnoses with breast cancer than those who never took an antibiotic.[117]

Why do kids get so many infections to which they are brought to doctors? It's their diet. Dr. Fuhrman tells story after story of kids who come to his office, chronically ill and amazingly he changes the family diet and no more sickness.

I have personally noticed that I have not had a bad cold since I stopped eating dairy over one year ago. I drive carpool and in the winter I hear the kids in my carpool trying to breathe through their clogged noses and coughing up so much mucus. I remember those days of feeling that way myself and how miserable it was. I don't miss that one bit!

"Let food be thy medicine and medicine be thy food." Hippocrates.

CHAPTER 29

WHAT ABOUT PESTICIDES?

THERE ARE SOME foods that are known to have even more chemicals than others. If you absolutely can't afford to buy organic, try your best to grow a garden. If you buy standard non-organic fruits and veggies, make sure to at least wash them with a really good organic fruit and veggie cleaner. Eating chemicals is never smart, but it's less carcinogenic than eating animal products and causes less disease than eating oils and processed foods.

EWG's 2016 Shopper's Guide to Pesticides in Produce [118]
Nearly three-fourths of the 6,953 produce samples tested by the U.S. Department of Agriculture in 2014 contained pesticide residues, a surprising finding in the face of soaring consumer demand for food without synthetic chemicals.

This year's update to the Environmental Working Group's Shopper's Guide to Pesticides in Produce™ reports that the USDA tests found a total 146 different pesticides on thousands of fruit and vegetable samples examined in 2014. The pesticides persisted on fruits and vegetables tested by the USDA, even when they were washed and, in some cases, peeled.

The USDA findings indicate that the conventional fruit and produce industries are ignoring a striking market trend: American consumers are voting with their pocketbooks for produce with less pesticide. Yet EWG's Shopper's Guide to Pesticides in Produce™ recognizes that many people who want to reduce their exposure to pesticides cannot find or afford an all-organic diet. The Guide helps consumers to identify conventionally grown fruits and vegetables that tend to test low on the scale for pesticide residues. When consumers want foods whose conventional versions test high for pesticides, they can make an effort to locate organic products.

Highlights of the "Dirty Dozen," 2016
EWG singles out produce with the highest pesticide loads for its "Dirty Dozen"™ list. This year, it includes strawberries, apples, nectarines, peaches, celery, grapes, cherries, spinach, tomatoes, sweet bell peppers, cherry tomatoes, and cucumbers.

Each of these foods tested positive for a number of different pesticide residues and showed higher concentrations of pesticides than other produce.

Key findings:

- More than 98 percent of strawberry samples, peaches, nectarines, and apples tested positive for at least one pesticide residue.
- The average potato had more pesticides by weight than any other produce.
- A single grape sample and a sweet bell pepper sample contained 15 pesticides.
- Single samples of strawberries showed 17 different pesticides.

The "Clean Fifteen"
EWG's "Clean Fifteen"™ list of the produce least likely to have pesticide residues consists of avocados, sweet corn, pineapples, cabbage, frozen sweet peas, onions, asparagus, mangoes, papayas, kiwis, eggplant, honeydew melon, grapefruit, cantaloupe, and cauliflower. Relatively few pesticides were detected on these foods, and tests found low total concentrations of pesticides on them.

Key findings:

- Avocados were the cleanest: only one percent of avocado samples showed any detectable pesticides.
- Some 89 percent of pineapples, 81 percent of papayas, 78 percent of mangoes, 73 percent of kiwis and 62 percent of cantaloupes had no residues.

- *No single fruit sample from the "Clean Fifteen"™ tested positive for more than four types of pesticides.*
- *Multiple pesticide residues are extremely rare on "Clean Fifteen"™ vegetables. Only five and a half percent of "Clean Fifteen" samples had two or more pesticides.*

The "Dirty Dozen Plus"

The EWG states that, for the fourth year, we have expanded the Dirty Dozen™ with a plus category to highlight two types of food that contain trace levels of highly hazardous pesticides. Leafy greens - kale and collard greens - and hot peppers do not meet traditional Dirty Dozen™ ranking criteria but were frequently found to be contaminated with insecticides toxic to the human nervous system. EWG recommends that people who eat a lot of these foods buy organic instead.

Leafy greens and hot peppers carry toxic pesticides.

Two American food crops - leafy greens and hot peppers - are of special concern for public health because residue tests conducted by the U.S. Department of Agriculture have found these foods laced with particularly toxic pesticides. Among the chemicals at issue are organophosphate and carbamate insecticides. These are no longer detected widely on other produce, either because of binding legal restrictions or voluntary phase-outs.

Leafy greens did not qualify for EWG's Dirty Dozen™ list this year under the traditional EWG Shopper's Guide rating system, which highlights produce with the highest number and concentrations of pesticides. Still, because of the extraordinary toxicity of the pesticides detected on them, we are highlighting them in this special Plus section.

USDA tests of 739 samples of hot peppers in 2010 and 2011 (USDA 2010, 2011) found residues of three highly toxic insecticides — acephate, chlorpyrifos, and oxamyl — on a portion of sampled peppers at concentrations high enough to cause concern. These insecticides are banned on some crops but still allowed on hot peppers.

In tests conducted in 2007 and 2008, USDA scientists detected 51 pesticides on kale and 41 pesticides on collard greens (USDA 2007, 2008).

Several of those pesticides — chlorpyrifos, famoxadone, oxydemeton, dieldrin, DDE and esfenvalerate — are highly toxic. Although many farmers may have changed their pesticide practices since 2008, chlorpyrifos and esfenvalerate are still permitted on leafy greens. Organochlorine pesticides DDE and dieldrin were banned some years ago but persist in agricultural soils and still make their way onto leafy greens grown today.

CHAPTER 30

BUY SOME KITCHEN GADGETS

A VERY GOOD investment at a very reasonable price is a pressure cooker. I know how busy we all are and spending hours in the kitchen is just not realistic, but a pressure cooker cuts cooking time in half or less! Last night I made a pasta dish in the pressure cooker that literally took 20 minutes, and that included prep time, cooking time (six minutes) and on plates to eat, and it was delicious! I also love my food processor for mixing hummus, chopping veggies and nuts; my blender for making nut milks, plant based milk shakes and sauces and my grain mill for making homemade organic flour. (I use Chef Brad's "WonderFlour[119]" recipe, which is equal parts of brown rice, spelt and barley.) A sharp knife is imperative, and lots of cutting boards are handy especially when you get the kids involved. Good cookware that does not leach chemicals into your food is a must! I've purchased all these items in the past year and I'm not sure how I lived without them before. Now I'm saving for a bread mixer. I'm so jealous of Chef Brad's bread rising in six minutes with his bread mixer while I watch my bread slowly rise on the counter! I did live without these kitchen tools for many, many years, so don't use a small budget and little to no kitchen gadgets as a reason to buy processed food for your kids. Do be prepared to spend a little extra time in the kitchen. Get your family involved. It's more fun when everyone is helping while spending quality time together and learning cooking skills. Remember your family's health is in your hands. You can do it!

CHAPTER 31

START COLLECTING YOUR FAVORITE RECIPES

RECIPE MAKING AND collecting is fun and delicious. But keep in mind that simple is just fine. You don't actually need recipes; they are just a bonus. You can make pasta with marinara sauce, mashed potatoes and gravy, bean burritos, rice and veggie stir fry, and bean, grain and veggie soups all pretty easily without a recipe. But if you want to fancy it up a bit, you can. Just be sure your recipes are animal free and oil free. You can replace meat with grains or starches. You can replace oil with apple sauce when baking. You can replace eggs with Ener-G egg replacer. I also use 100% pure organic maple syrup instead of sugar. But even easier, you can google plant based oil free recipes and find lots of great ones. I recently found Jill McKeever[120] on YouTube being fun and silly while cooking quick and healthy recipes for her family. With the technology available today the information we can access is limitless.

I also like *The China Study Cookbook*, the *Prevent and Reverse Heart Disease Cookbook* and the *Plant Based Families Cookbook*. But even more, I like making my own recipes and sharing them with you. Check out a few simple favorites at the end of this book, or on my blog at www.NourishAndStrengthen.org[121], or my Facebook page at www.facebook.com/nourishAndStrengthen[122]

CHAPTER 32

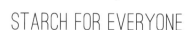

STARCH FOR EVERYONE

I ENJOYED LISTENING to a great lecture about why we should eat starch for our main food by Dr. McDougall.[123] My favorite line of his from this webinar was, "Your health is trying to get out of you, stop poisoning yourself so it can!"

Here are the reasons you should eat starches and not animals according to Dr. McDougall.

1. Starches are easy to grow, such as corn, rice, potatoes, etc.
2. Starches are inexpensive to buy, such as beans, rice, corn, and oats.
3. Starches are high energy. Ask any athlete and they know to eat starches (aka carbs) before the race or big game.
4. Starches are complete nutrition. They have calcium, fat, vitamins, fiber, protein, and no cholesterol. Starches do not have the B12 bacteria found in animals, so do take vitamin B12 if you are animal free for more than three years just to be safe. Potatoes and sweet potatoes have ALL the nutrition you need to survive. Grains are a close second, just add a bit of A and C vitamins in the form of an orange or broccoli if you want to live on grains only.
5. Animals are full of deadly chemicals.
6. Have you seen videos of animals being raised for the slaughter or providing us with milk and milk products? Have a conscience!

7. Save the Earth with starches. You can grow an average of 17 times more calories on the same amount of land as you can animal products. Switching from beef to potatoes is 100 times!
8. Starches don't grow germs and diseases. If your starches or fruit or veggies are infected, it came from an animal or a human.
9. Starches taste good! Sweet potatoes, corn, potatoes, etc.—our taste buds are made for sugar. That's why we like starches so much!
10. Starches store well. How long can you store grains? Forever!
11. Starches are easy to travel with.
12. Starches are great for weight loss. They are filling yet very low in fat and calories. Potatoes are one percent fat and that's all your body needs!
13. All starches are created equal. Choose one or two or more and stick to them. There is no one "best" starch.
14. The author of the *Blue Zones*[124] realized when speaking to Dr. McDougall that the key to what makes people live the longest is eating starches!
15. It's really hard for your body to convert starch to fat. Look at all the thin Asians who eat rice and veggies! They don't gain weight until they try our American diet.

To have the ultimate health and ideal weight, you need lots of starches, some fruits and veggies, B12, sunshine and a walk. Simple![125]

CHAPTER 33

CAN YOU MAKE THAT?

WHAT CAN YOU make instead of buy? Make your favorite foods free of animal products, oils and chemicals!

Here are a few ideas:

Popcorn
Hot Cocoa
Soups
Bread
Nut Milk
Nut Cheese
Oil-Free Dips/Sauces/Dressings
Tortilla Chips
Ice Cream
Cakes
Pizza
Hummus
Smoothies

The list is endless! What can you add?

For an endless list of oil free plant based recipes, visit: https://www.drmcdougall.com/health/education/recipes/mcdougall-newsletter-recipes/.[126]

CHAPTER 34

SUGAR IS NOT THE ENEMY

Is sugar good for you? No! Is it the worst thing for you? No! It's the perfect storm that Americans eat. They eat meat and dairy which causes tumor growth, and then they eat sugar and more animal products and refined foods and oils and chemicals which feed the growth. Cancer usually doubles in size every 100 days. Do you want to eat food that grows cancer or food that starves cancer?

God made us the perfect desserts. We have fruits and nuts and even maple syrup. As you start eating a whole food, plant based diet, natural desserts will satisfy your taste buds and keep you feeling wonderful.

Is it terrible to sprinkle a bit of sugar on your plant based desserts or oatmeal? No. When choosing a sugar, the less refined the better. And, a little bit goes a long way!

Please remember that animal products are worse for you than sugar!

To put that in perspective, read what John McDougall MD has written about sugar.

We Are Hard-Wired to Enjoy Sugar[127]
Humans are anatomically and physiologically designed to seek and consume sugar. The tip of our tongue tastes with pleasure only one calorie-containing substance, sugar (carbohydrate). In our natural environment this stimulus comes from plant foods—such as, potatoes, sweet potatoes, beans, rice, fruits, and vegetables. Food manufacturers take advantage of our nature, adding highly-refined, powerful-tasting sugars to our foods.

Once past the tongue, the remainder of the intestinal tract, as well as all of the internal systems of the body, is geared to efficiently utilize sugars. Our nervous system uses sugars almost exclusively as a source of energy—and 20% of the calories consumed daily go to operate the brain.

Research indicates that consumption of carbohydrates provides a reward to the person by producing opioid- and dopamine-mediated responses—changes in the brain's chemistry which cause us to feel pleasure. The sweet taste of sugar produces intense pleasure with effects similar to those derived from the use of narcotics (opium). Therefore, us "pleasure seekers" quickly learn from our tongues and our brains that consuming carbohydrate is the right thing to do—and consuming sugar is intoxicating.

Some tissues of our body, such as red blood cells and kidney cells (glomeruli cells) will only burn carbohydrates. Endurance athletes know well the winning advantage of a diet high in sugars (carbohydrates)—sports drinks used during their races are made of concentrated simple sugars. Considering the importance of sugars to our existence, why are they vilified? Before discussing some of the negative consequences of consuming too much refined sugar, I need to clear up some important misinformation.

The Human Body Does Not Turn Sugar to Fat

The process of synthesizing fat from sugar is known as de novo lipogenesis—the new production of fat. This activity is highly efficient in some animals, such as pigs and cows—which is one reason they have become popular people foods—these animals can convert low-energy, inexpensive carbohydrates—grass, say, in the case of cows and grains for pigs—into calorie-dense fats. However, human beings are very inefficient at this process and as a result de novo lipogenesis does not occur under usual living conditions in people. Thus the common belief that sugar turns to fat is scientifically incorrect—and there is no disagreement about this fact among scientists or their scientific research.

*Under experimental laboratory conditions, however, where people are **overfed large amounts of simple sugars**, the human body will resort to converting a small amount of sugar into a small amount of fat (triglycerides) in the liver. For example, in one recent study, trim and obese women were overfed with 50%*

more calories than they usually ate—note, 535 of these extra calories each day came from four and a half ounces (135 grams) of refined sugar. In this forced-fed situation, the women produced less than 4 grams (36 calories) of fat daily from the extra carbohydrate. Extrapolation from these findings means a person would have to be overfed by this amount of food and table sugar every day for nearly 4 months in order to gain one extra pound of body fat from the conversion of sugar to fat—by de novo lipogenesis. Obviously, even overeating substantial quantities of sugar is a relatively unimportant source of body fat. (So where does all that fat come from? The fat you eat is the fat you wear.)

Sugar Does Not Cause Obesity
A universally accepted mantra among dieters is, "Don't eat starches—starches turn to sugar—sugar makes you fat." If this were true then obesity would be rampant among rice-eating Japanese—obviously, the opposite is the case. Worldwide, populations with the highest consumption of carbohydrate are the trimmest and fittest.

Studies of people also show that the higher their sugar intake the lower their calorie intake and the fewer people who are overweight. This makes a lot of sense because when you add carbohydrate (even pure sugar) to the diet then fat must be removed—kind of a fat-sugar seesaw—one goes up, then the other must go down. Fat is very concentrated in calories (9 per gram vs. 4 for pure sugar), fat is almost effortlessly stored, and fat provides little appetite satisfaction. Thus, replacing fat in the diet with sugar will cause weight loss. Furthermore, the practice by "low-carbohydrate dieters" of decreasing sugar intake often results in a higher calorie intake, because of all the fat that is added.

Sugar Does Not Cause Diabetes
After eating high-carbohydrate foods you might suspect that all that dietary sugar would cause the sugar in the blood to rise and this might lead to diabetes. That's what many lay people believe. Even a few scientists have theorized that chronically elevated levels of sugar in the blood might wear out the insulin-producing cells of the pancreas and produce diabetes. Actually, this common thinking is incorrect—studies comparing sugar intake with risk of developing type-2

diabetes show people on high sugar diets are less likely to get diabetes. There is, however, a strong relationship between red meat consumption and diabetes.

The lowest rates of diabetes in the world are found among populations that consume the most carbohydrate—for this reason type-2 diabetes is almost unknown in rural Asia, Africa, Mexico and Peru. However, when these people change to a diet rich in fats and low in carbohydrates they commonly become diabetic. Some of the highest rates of this disease (and associated obesity) are found in Hispanics, Native Americans, Polynesians, and Blacks who have recently adopted the American diet.

Contrary to popular belief, refined sugars actually make the body's insulin work more efficiently. When the refined sugar content of an experimental diet of people with mild diabetes was doubled from 45% sugar to 85% sugar, every measurement of their diabetic condition improved—fasting blood sugar, fasting insulin levels, and the oral glucose tolerance test all showed their diabetes was better. The researchers concluded, "These data suggest that the high carbohydrate diet increased the sensitivity of peripheral tissues to insulin." The increase in insulin's sensitivity (efficiency) exceeds any blood sugar-raising effect from consuming more carbohydrate. Because sugar does not cause type-2 diabetes, the American Diabetic Association has recommended "55% to 65% of a diabetic's diet come from carbohydrate," and sugary foods are allowed.

The carbohydrates found in whole foods (starches, vegetables, and fruits) are much healthier to consume than refined sugars for a person wanting to prevent or cure type-2 diabetes for a variety of reasons—especially because of the adverse effects on weight gain and blood cholesterol and triglycerides of sugars compared to starches (more in next month's newsletter). A high carbohydrate, vegan diet, has recently been shown to help diabetics stop medications and improve their overall health.

Acceptable Sugar Use

The main reason sugar has a bad reputation is because of the company it keeps. People living in Western societies eat loads of rich foods that make them fat and sick. Along with their high intake of meat, dairy, and refined grains, they also eat a lot of simple sugars. In this cauldron of malnutrition, sugar's exact *contribution becomes indistinct. But, in most people's minds, sugar is the villain—the scapegoat, taking focus off the animal-foods and free fats (vegetable oils), which are much more of a burden to one's health than simple sugar is. This misplaced emphasis results in a lost opportunity to regain lost health and appearance.*

Sugar tastes great and can hugely enhance the enjoyment of eating. One practical point is that the addition of sugar will boost the acceptance of a low-fat diet, like the McDougall diet—increasing long-term compliance. However, to reap the greatest pleasure with the least harm, simple sugar should be put on the surface of the food where the tongue makes direct contact. This means sugars should not be added to the food during preparation—mixed up in the ingredients where the sweet flavors are hidden from the tongue's taste buds. Using a small amount of sugar on the surface of the food is my recommendation for trim, healthy people.

However, there can be some real drawbacks and health hazards caused by consuming simple sugars, especially for those in poor health. If you have concerns about your weight loss or have artery (heart) disease, then you should strictly limit your intake of all simple sugars, including fruits and their juices.

CHAPTER 35

USDA DIETARY GUIDELINES FOR AMERICANS 2015-2020

TIP NUMBER ONE. Don't get your nutrition facts from the government! Why? The USDA was formed to help agribusiness. Many of the members of the USDA are from the egg, meat and dairy industries. They are trying to sell a product, not trying to help us be healthier.

I had the treat of listening to Dr. McDougall discuss this new guideline[128] which he and some other California physicians along with the Physicians Committee of Responsible Medicine, are suing the USDA over. They feel the new guideline is a threat to American health and keeps their patients sick.[129] Here are some of the notes I took while listening to Dr. McDougall mixed with my commentary.

Who follows the USDA guidelines? 300 million children eating school lunches and all public nutrition programs to name a few! For the big industries to sell their product yet make us think they are helping us out, they make the guidelines confusing and contradictory. For example, they say eat vegetables, fruits and grains, great! But then they add: eat dairy, meat, seafood and oils, which are terrible for your health. Then they say sugar, saturated fat, salt and alcohol are bad. Then they recommend foods high in these ingredients like yogurt, meat and cheese. These foods are full of sugar, saturated fat and sodium. The guideline says legumes are good for protein as well as seafood and meat. Then they outline the benefits, listing vitamins and fiber, and make you think they are talking about the meat when they are actually talking about the legumes.

The guideline conveniently forgets to mention to be cautious of infectious diseases and contaminants found in meat. They list vitamins and proteins and make it sound like we have a great risk of becoming deficient. Yet there has never in the world been a protein deficiency for anyone who ate enough calories of anything. Even the seven decade Kempner rice study at Duke University[130] with 5% protein content did not give anyone protein deficiencies. Not only that, the rice diet healed almost every one of their chronic diseases—wow!

Some people are low on vitamin D because they don't get any sunlight and they eat animal products that block vitamin D absorption. The guideline mentions all the nutrition that comes from dairy. Don't forget, Americans are not short on nutrition; quite the contrary. The guideline forgets to mention that dairy is the main cause of allergies and autoimmune disease. Did you know that milk is high in saturated fat, trans fats, chemicals, microbes, and is the most recalled food item? They forgot to mention that too! You hear of vegetable contamination on the news, and the media makes a big deal of dangerous cucumbers or strawberries etc.; here is the actual news. For veggies to get contaminated they have to touch human or animal poop. Veggies are not contaminated like animal products are.

The guideline says you need EPA and DHA and tells you to eat seafood, but then says beware of methyl-mercury which comes from where? You guessed it, seafood! The guideline says to get your essential fatty acids, but all studies show that when you increase your fatty acids you increase your heart disease. Oops, forgot to mention that too. Not a big deal though, because only 1 in 2 men and 1 in 3 women in American die from heart disease!

Then the USDA reminds us to not eat saturated fat, but do eat the products containing them in the highest quantities, meat, poultry, dairy and eggs. The big industries were happy to get the cholesterol limit out of the guideline this time around as one egg contains 247 mg of cholesterol. How can you eat meat all day (cholesterol) when you've already met your daily limit with your one egg at breakfast, right? And there is no limit on fat intake either. Yippee. Oh wait, half of Americans are suffering with chronic diseases, obesity costs

Americans $147 billion per year with two-thirds of adults being obese and one-third of kids, and we spend $245 billion on diabetes per year. Did you know that you can cure type 2 diabetes in about 10 days by eating a whole food, plant based diet?

The egg industry spends $23 million per year to convince you to eat eggs. The facts are pretty simple. When your cholesterol is up, so is your risk of heart disease. Did you know that of the six major studies on eggs and their effect on people, five of them were done by the egg industry? And they only allow us to see the studies done after 2003. A trick they use to help their numbers is to only allow those people with extremely high cholesterol to participate in their studies. A person who is already soaked in cholesterol can't absorb a whole lot more and the result looks as if the cholesterol from the egg is not affecting the people studied very much. Try feeding an egg to a person with low cholesterol and see what happens; their cholesterol jumps by large amounts. These are the reports your nutritionist is getting handed to them—studies that make the product (an egg in this example) look like it's not so bad. No wonder everyone is so confused.

Last but not least, if you don't care about yourself or your health, how about saving the land, the water and the animals from cruel treatment? Something's got to give. I'm anxious to see how this lawsuit plays out, and I hope you think twice before you put animal products into your body.

CHAPTER 36

MAKE YOUR OWN BABY FOOD

WHY MAKE YOUR own baby food when you can buy it at the store? Imagine that precious little baby that you want to love and protect and keep safe no matter what the cost. You nurse the baby until the baby is ready for food and then what do you put inside the baby? Hopefully, not pesticides and processed foods! Instead, nourish and strengthen the baby; do not feed the baby processed food or non-organic food. Does it take extra time and effort to make baby food? Of course it does. But isn't your baby or grand-baby worth it?

Take a potato or a sweet potato, a squash or some peas, etc. Buy them organic or grow them organically in your garden. Steam them on your kitchen stove in a strainer basket with hot water underneath. Keep those nutrients in the food as much as you can by not overcooking. Then throw the steamed potato or sweet potato etc. in the blender with some filtered water and puree it. Put the baby food in glass jars in your refrigerator. Or boil them and make them airtight and keep them in your pantry. Your baby deserves the best start, the best health, and nothing that would damage the baby's body should go inside the baby.

After reading learning about "the dirty dozen," I've decided that I will make baby food for my grandkids when I have them! What a perfect gift from a grandma to her grandkids. I may have to freeze it and ship it across the country, but I will do that if necessary!

You hear about kids getting cancer and it breaks my heart. Typically, it takes a lifetime of food abuse to create disease in our bodies, but some kids have weaker systems and fall prey to cell mutations sooner than most of us. If we can avoid animal products and feed our children pesticide-free food and whole foods that are not processed, and use natural soaps and cleaners, our children and families have the best chance for good health. It's so worth our time and effort!

Remember however, that according to Colin T. Campbell,[131] casein, or milk protein, is the most carcinogenic food every found. Dr. Campbell says this in almost every speech he gives. Please don't feed your baby pesticide free, plant based food and then give them animal products that are found to cause tumor growth. Let's keep our kids healthy and disease free.

CHAPTER 37

DRINK FILTERED WATER

IS IT REALLY that big of a deal to drink filtered water? Tap water doesn't taste that bad to some people. Is it really just taste we are concerned about? As with our food, our concern needs to run much deeper than taste alone.

Water is a life-sustaining fluid that's essential to health, but if you're drinking straight out of the tap, it can undermine your health. When you drink tap (or even spring) water, you'll likely be getting more than you bargained for—chlorine, fluorine compounds, trihalomethanes (THMs), assorted hormones, pesticides and even trace amounts of prescription drugs.

It can be a witches' brew of health-killing effluvia, but you can improve the odds. Here's the lowdown on water, and how to turn it back into the health drink nature intended.

Tap water is dirtier than it looks

Even "clean" drinking water that flows from the tap isn't what most of us would think of as clean. It's traveled through miles of pipeline, picking up contaminants, pesticides and industrial run-off along the way. It's been disinfected with potential carcinogens like chlorine, ammonia and or chloramines, then "fortified" with fluoride. While disinfection is a necessary evil—without it, waterborne illnesses would be a constant problem—drinking, showering and bathing every day with this chemical brew is a lousy idea.

No. Seriously. Your water is funky

The problem is, most of us don't have a clue about the chemicals and contaminants in our water, nor do we know their long-term effects. We trust that everything is ok, but it's not. In fact, the Environmental Working Group spent three years investigating the country's drinking water and the results were jaw-dropping. They found that roughly 85% of the population was using tap water laced with over 300 contaminants, many with unknown long-term effects, and more than half of which aren't even regulated by the EPA. Add to the mix an ever-growing list of new chemical compounds that become available just about every day and well, the waters only get murkier.

Bottled water isn't better, cleaner, or good for the earth

Let me be blunt: there's just no good reason to drink bottled water — and if you're one of those folks who buys it by the case, I beg you to stop. Bottled water is virtually unregulated, expensive, and even the EPA says it's not necessarily safer than tap. It's also insanely wasteful — an estimated three liters of water is needed to produce just one liter, and roughly 17 million barrels of oil is required to produce all those bottles, according to The Pacific Institute. What's worse, roughly two-thirds of those bottles wind up in the ocean and in landfills, polluting and poisoning waters and wildlife.

Brew your own with the help of water filtration systems

So, how to reduce the bad stuff in your brew? The best way to go is to use a water filtration system. For starters, look for one that's certified by the NSF, an independent, non-profit group that tests and verifies the contaminant reducing abilities of water filters. Next, you'll need to determine how far you're willing to go based on your needs and budget. Ideally, whole-house filtration systems are an excellent option, but they're not always feasible. If whole-house filtration isn't appropriate for your home, I recommend investing in individual drinking water and shower filter units.

Tap into your tap. For drinking water, there are different ways to go, with the three simplest options being under-the-counter filters, countertop filters and pitcher systems.

Under-the-counter systems are great because they're tucked away out of sight and receive very high marks for filtration. However, the initial purchase price plus the usage cost per gallon can be a bit higher than the other options, and there is some installation involved.

Countertop filters use water pressure to force water through the filtration process, which helps to make water healthier and tastier, and removing more contaminants than standard pitcher systems. Countertop systems require minimal installation (a small hose, but no permanent fixtures) and take up only few inches of counter space.

Water pitchers work well for the space-challenged because they're portable, need no installation, fit easily in the fridge and are available on just about every street corner. They do a decent job of filtering out some of the major contaminants, but generally not as many as under-the-counter and countertop versions. And while the initial investment is small, filters need frequent replacement, which boosts the cost per gallon over other methods. My favorite pitcher (and the one we use in my office) is the Aquasana Powered Water Filtration System.

Don't bathe in chemicals

Your morning shower should not include daily exposure to chlorine, carcinogens and vaporized chemical contaminants being absorbed into your skin and breathed into your lungs. Without a shower filter, it does.

Here's a few simple tips to cut exposure:

- Shorten your showers.
- Turn down the temperature a bit so your skin pores are less open for absorbing contaminants.
- Install a shower filter (most important).[132]

CHAPTER 38

EAT SPROUTS!

I HOPE YOU will make or buy some sprouts to enjoy on your salads, sandwiches and more. They are really fun and easy to grow in your kitchen too. Buy a sprout growing kit and learn how easy and nutritious it can be.

The health benefits of sprouts make up quite an impressive list, and they include the ability to improve the digestive process, boost the metabolism, increase enzymatic activity throughout the body, prevent anemia, help with weight loss, lower cholesterol, reduce blood pressure, prevent neural tube defects in infants, protect against cancer, boost skin health, improve vision, support the immune system, and increase usable energy reserves.

Sprouts may refer to a number of different vegetable or plant beans in the period of time after they begin to grow. The most common sprouts that people regularly use in cooking are alfalfa, soy, and mung bean sprouts, as well as various other types of bean sprouts. The reason that so many people turn to sprouts as a source of food is that they represent a much more significant amount of vitamins and nutrients than they do in an un-sprouted form. Typically, a week after sprouting, the sprouts will have the highest concentration and bioavailability of nutrients. Beans must contain a packed storehouse of all the important nutrients that a plant will need to grow in its initial days, so those tiny caps are filled with important organic compounds, vitamins, and minerals that our body can also utilize.

There are a number of different cultures that highly value sprouts as an essential element of their cooking. Although sprouts can be cultivated anywhere that beans are grown (which is basically anywhere in the world), Asian nations seem to have adopted sprouts as a topping for various dishes, as well as a common ingredient in salads more than most other countries in the world. They are readily available no matter what market you go to, however.

The important thing to remember is that much of the nutritive value of sprouts is lost when they are heated. In other words, although they are a very important source of nutrients and beneficial health boosts, they should always be added to meal in their raw form to guarantee that they have the most impact. Let's explore some of the components of sprouts that make them such a powerful, yet overlooked, source of so many health benefits.

Nutritional Value of Sprouts

All of the nutritional and medicinal benefits of sprouts are derived from their impressive vitamin, mineral, and organic compounds content. Sprouts contain a significant amount of protein and dietary fiber, as well as vitamin K, folate, pantothenic acid, niacin, thiamin, vitamin C, vitamin A, and riboflavin. In terms of minerals, sprouts contain manganese, copper, zinc, magnesium, iron, and calcium. Many of these component nutrients increase dramatically as the sprout continues to develop. Along with all of those components, sprouts are also a rich source of enzymes that are essential for health. It is best to eat sprouts that first opened one or two weeks earlier. Now, let's explore some of the fascinating and vital health benefits that sprouts hold for us!

Health Benefits of Sprouts

Digestion: One of the best things about sprouts is that they contain an unusually high number of enzymes. This can help boost the various metabolic processes and chemical reactions within the body, specifically when it comes to digestion. Enzymes are an important part of the digestive process, and they help to break down food effectively and increase the absorption of nutrients by the digestive tract. Furthermore, the dietary fiber found in sprouts makes it a very important boost for digestive functions. Fiber bulks up the stool, making it easier to pass through the digestive tract. Furthermore, dietary fiber stimulates gastric juices, which aid the enzymes already found in sprouts in breaking down food effectively and efficiently. Sprouts are a great way to clear up constipation, as well as diarrhea, and can even prevent colorectal cancer.

Metabolic Booster
As was already mentioned, sprouts contain a wealth of enzymes that usually aren't available through food. This major influx represents a kick start for the body, and can seriously impact the metabolic activity of your body. Beyond that, sprouts also contain a significant amount of protein, which is the essential part of food that allows our body to perform all of its chemical functions. Protein is necessary for almost all bodily processes, particularly the creation and maintenance of cells, organ repair, skin regeneration, bone growth, muscle development, and a number of other very important aspects of health. This means that sprouts are an easy and delicious way to improve the overall functioning and development of your body.

Anemia and Blood Circulation
Anemia is the technical word for an iron deficiency. If you don't consume enough food with iron, your red blood cell count drops, because iron is an essential part of red blood cell production. This can result in fatigue, lack of concentration, nausea, light-headedness, and stomach disorders. By maintaining your red blood cell count with proper amounts of iron (and copper, which is also found in sprouts), you can improve the circulation of blood in your body, thereby increasing the oxygenation of organ systems and cells to optimize their performance.

Weight Loss
Sprouts are one of those foods that are very high in nutrients but very low in calories. This means that you can eat sprouts without worrying about compromising your diet. Furthermore, the fiber in sprouts helps to make you feel full, both by adding bulk to your bowels, but also by inhibiting the release of ghrelin, which is the hunger hormone that tells our mind that we are ready to eat something. This can reduce overeating and snacking, two of the biggest problems for someone suffering through the problems of obesity.

Heart Health
Sprouts are a great source of omega-3 fatty acids, and although these are technically a form of cholesterol, they are considered "good" cholesterol (HDL

cholesterol) and can actually reduce the amount of harmful cholesterol in your blood vessels and arteries. Omega-3 fatty acids are also anti-inflammatory in nature, so they reduce the stress on your cardiovascular system in that was as well. The potassium content of sprouts also helps to reduce blood pressure, since potassium is a vasodilator, and can release the tension in arteries and blood vessels. This increases circulation and oxygenation, while reducing clotting and lowering the risk of atherosclerosis, heart attacks, and strokes.

Infant Health
Neural tube defects are one of the most common side effects of a deficiency in folate, a member of the B vitamin complex. Sprouts have a significant amount of folate, thereby protecting your infant from this tragic condition.

Immune System
There are a number of factors that make sprouts a powerful booster for the immune system. Its vitamin C content alone makes it a powerful stimulant for the white blood cells in the body to fight off infection and disease. Furthermore, as a sprout continues to develop, vitamin A can multiply almost ten times its original content. Vitamin A has a number of antioxidant properties that make a great source of immune system strength.

Cancer Prevention
The antioxidant activity of the organic compounds found in sprouts make it a very good anti-cancer choice for your diet. The vitamin C, vitamin A, as well as amino acids and proteins (including the huge amount of enzymes) can also impact the free radical content in the body. Free radicals are the natural, dangerous byproducts of cellular metabolism that can cause healthy cells to mutate into cancerous cells. They are also responsible for some heart diseases, premature aging, cognitive decline, and a variety of age-related health concerns. Sprouts can counteract these effects, thereby helping to reduce the chances of developing cancer.

Vision and Eye Health
Vitamin A has been associated with an improvement in vision health for many years. It acts as an antioxidant agent to protect the eyes' cells from free radicals.

In this way, sprouts can help prevent glaucoma, cataracts, and macular degeneration. In fact, vision can even improve in some cases, so eat your sprouts and start seeing the world a bit more clearly!

Cold Sores
Cold sores can be an unsightly, painful, and uncomfortable condition to suffer through. If they get infected, they can even become a serious health risk. There is a specific enzyme, called lysine, that actually inhibits the growth of cold sores and treats them if they do appear. This enzyme is conveniently found in significant amounts in sprouts!

Allergy and Asthma
Some varieties of sprouts, like broccoli sprouts, have been linked to reducing allergic reactions, including asthma, which is an inflammatory condition of the respiratory system. Although the exact chemical pathway is not fully understood, additional research is being done on this topic all the time.[133]

CHAPTER 39

MY KIDS WON'T EAT THAT

ACTUALLY THEY WILL! If you only have whole food, plant based dishes in your home, the kids will get hungry and they will eat it. This does not mean they will love eating plant based food on the first try, or they won't complain about it. Remember, if you don't start this from birth there will be a "learning curve" for the whole family, but that's okay. Changing your palate and your food addictions takes time, so be patient with yourself and your family. Look at the long run and the big picture and stick to it! It takes kids 8-15 tries before they like a new food. If you are like me, I used to give up after the third try feeding my kids something new and go for something sure to please them. There are foods my kids said they "HATED" and they would not go near but now, I have to smile as I watch them "LOVE" those same foods.

Change takes time. Give yourself lots of time. We all love change right? Wrong! We seem to be especially stubborn when it comes to our food. I think it's best to move slow and easy when changing the family diet. Remember, you are feeding your family this way to save them from disease and suffering and death. You're also saving the Earth, and the animals on it, the water and the air. Lately, in our house, I only have one child who complains and the rest are pretty happy to eat the yummy food I make them. Some even love it! When they are not at home I let them choose what they eat, but I hope that what I've taught them makes them think twice about their food choices. Some of my kids make good food choices away from home and others don't. I'm okay with that. We all have our agency and force is not a good plan.

Is the Standard American Diet (SAD diet) really that bad? Everybody around me eats the same way! Exactly! Eating the Standard American Diet is why almost everybody in America dies of disease instead of old age. As my friend Kelli always reminds me, parenting is not about taking the easy route. It's about doing what's best for your kids even when it's hard. I'm not saying to be a food tyrant. Give them choices. Let the kids help you garden, cook and learn about healthy eating. A great way to share healthy eating information with your family is by watching movies that are entertaining yet teach about health. Check out my favorite movie choices in Chapter 51, Family Movie Night or my family movie night blog post[134] (http://nourishandstrengthen.org/family-movie-night/). These movies have made a bigger impact on our food choices than anything else I have done.

It's important to teach your children not to be judgmental about other peoples' food choices. It's hard to convert others to healthy eating if you are teasing them or telling them they are wrong. Most people don't know that animal proteins cause disease, and since they are taught from a young age that animal proteins are good for them, they believe it. Lead by example, and encourage your children to share what they've learned in a kind manner if others are interested.

It's very rewarding when people love my whole food, plant based cooking. We had a birthday party at our house and I had a big grin as I watched all the teenagers devour my plant based food. I got an even bigger grin while watching them all come back for seconds. And an even bigger grin when my daughter came home from school a few days later and said her friends were wishing they had my food for their school lunches. Success!

CHAPTER 40

FOOD COLOR

THERE IS A reason that mint chip ice cream is green, and it's not because of the mint leaves. Remember, food companies are in the moneymaking business. The better it tastes, the more addictive it is, and the prettier it looks means that you will buy more. But what are those dyes doing to your body besides turning your tongue bright colors? Ask any parent who has noticed that their child has sensitivities to dyes. They get hyper, crabby, mean, and downright crazy, to name a few symptoms. But those are just obvious outward symptoms. What happens to your insides?

Carmine, also referred to as cochineal extract or natural red 4, comes from dried bugs. It has been used in food since the 16th century. Only recently has research linked it to anaphylactic shock.

FD&C yellow #5, also referred to as tartrazine, is one of two yellow food dyes that has been associated with allergic reactions. People have reported hives and swelling after eating foods containing FD&C yellow #5. Studies many years ago also suggested tartrazine might trigger asthma attacks in children, although recent research hasn't found the same evidence.

Annatto, the other yellow dye, annatto, comes from the seeds of the achiote tree, which is found in tropical countries. Annatto gives foods a yellow-orange color. Studies have reported several cases of severe, anaphylactic reactions in people who were sensitive to this dye.

The symptoms of a food dye reaction can be mild or severe. During a mild reaction, you might notice:

flushing, headaches, hives, itchy skin, swelling of the face.

A severe reaction may include:

tightness in the chest, difficulty breathing, or wheezing, dizziness or fainting, fast heartbeat, low blood pressure, tightness in your throat, and trouble breathing.

If you develop severe symptoms, call 911 immediately. This reaction can be life threatening.

If you know that you have a severe food dye allergy, you should carry around an epinephrine auto-injector at all times. An auto-injector is considered the first-line treatment for a severe food allergy reaction."[135]

Or better yet, eat the colors that nature made and avoid negative reactions in your body.

CHAPTER 41

BREASTFEEDING

BREAST FEED YOUR babies for as long as you both can take it. Within reason of course! Like that movie Grown Ups,[136] Salma Hayek sees a friend's wife nursing their son and asks, "How old is he?" to which the father, Kevin James, replies "48 months," and his friend, Chris Rock, says, "that's four!" Or my daughter Ashley, who was nursing about every three to four hours; but then at seven months old, she woke up for her morning nursing and when I tried to feed her, she looked at me as if to say, "what kind of sicko are you?" and squirmed to get away from me. And that was that, she never nursed again! What is within reason? That's up to mommy and baby but try not to be so anxious to give it up; it's the perfect food for the health for your baby. When our oldest child turned one year old we started letting her drink cow's milk and that's when she began to have a chronically stuffy and tickly nose, but we didn't put two and two together. She also quickly developed a lot of other allergies. She is our only child with allergies. She is allergic to dogs, cats, eggs, almonds, cashews, pistachios, dairy and wheat. Oh my! I'm convinced that it was because of the milk she drank at a young age. Sorry, Bekah. I didn't know.

"An infant allergy to cow's milk may show up as soon as the parent introduces formula, because about 80 percent of formulas are milk-based. Up to 7.5 percent of infants can develop this allergy. So how will you know if your child is one of them? Symptoms of child or infant food allergies may include skin rashes, hives, wheezing, nasal congestion, and digestive problems," Heidi Renner, MD, notes.[137]"

According to the Mayo Clinic, *Milk allergy symptoms, which differ from person to person, occur a few minutes to a few hours after drinking milk or eating milk products.*

Immediately after consuming milk, signs and symptoms of a milk allergy might include:

Hives
Wheezing
Vomiting

Signs and symptoms that may take more time to develop include:

Loose stools, which may contain blood
Diarrhea
Abdominal cramps
Coughing or wheezing
Runny nose
Watery eyes
Itchy skin rash, often around the mouth
Colic, in babies[138]

Many baby formulas are made with a cow's milk base. Why chance these symptoms with your sweet baby? If mom is eating lots of dairy and nursing, her baby can have reactions too. Let's avoid dairy.

You don't want to use baby formula either because of the terrible ingredients in baby formula. I heard the other day that the first ingredient in a certain baby formula was corn syrup. Need I say more? That is so sad. Our bodies are made to care for our young and nourish them. Let's take advantage of this great blessing and bonding time with our babies, for their health and ours.

CHAPTER 42

PARTY LIKE A WHOLE FOOD ROCK STAR!

THAT MEANS, EAT before you go to a party. Or better yet, bring something to share that you can eat! Food that adds health to your body and to those you share with. Plant based food is nutritious, delicious and beautiful so be ready to share the recipe. I LOVE it when people ask for the recipes of my whole food, plant based pot luck dishes. Success! If you go to a party starving and there are not many healthy choices, it's going to be hard to make the right decisions, so plan ahead.

Vegan foods are not a good choice either. The average vegan eats a 30% fat diet. A plant based diet contains 6-10% fat. Remember that a gram of fat has nine calories and a gram of starches/carbohydrates has four calories. That means you can eat more than twice as much food for the same calorie count by eating starches instead of fat. We are not talking about counting calories here; I just wanted to help you to see why it's harder to gain weight eating starches. Of course health is the goal, but low body weight and feeling great are side benefits.

Don't cheat! The reason I say this is because it leads down the wrong path. Going from the SAD (Standard American Diet) diet to a plant based diet is like giving up smoking. Once you are off the cigarettes, you feel good to be over the addiction and happy to regain your health. Those around you appreciate it too! So cheating on this diet is like going back to cigarettes. You might get the taste for them again, and then have to go through the whole exit process again. To me, it's not worth the health or addiction risk.

There are so many great party foods. Try one of these http://blog.fatfreevegan.com/category/appetizers-and-dips.[139]

CHAPTER 43

BROWN BAGGING IT

PACK YOUR KIDS' school lunch and yours too. Do you know who promotes their food in the school lunch program? Can you say Agribusiness? It's crazy that not only are our children given unhealthy food at school but they are told it's good for them. We've all heard that you need meat for protein and milk for calcium and oils for brain health, but it's not true. Why do most people believe these falsehoods? Who taught us this? Turn on your TV or open a magazine. The ones telling us this are the same ones making money from it—lots and lots of money. Beyond the animal proteins and oils, school lunches are processed foods full of preservatives. Are there whole food, plant based choices that are filling and will sustain a child through the day in the school cafeteria? Unlikely, unless you can live on carrot sticks.

Schools say that lunches are getting "better," but what does that mean? For me, in San Diego, schools say they are using better quality meat and buying more food locally. The problem is, animal protein causes tumor growth, heart disease and diabetes, to name a few. Is better quality disease causing food better? NO! Because they buy it local is it less disease causing? NO! Let's remember where the real problems lie: #1 is animal proteins of any type and #2 is processed foods/oils. So are school lunches really better? NO!

Decide how strict you are going to be with your kids about school lunch. Three of my kids are happy to eat what I pack for them and one, not so much. Not because it's not tasty, but because he's not into mom controlling his life. So with him, at this current time, I let him choose if he buys his lunch or I pack his lunch each day. I want to love him, not control him, so I give him the choice. It's so hard for me to do this. I know what the American diet does to our bodies. You'll have to discuss with your family what their choices are. The best way to influence their choices is by teaching them about health. See Chapter 51, Family Movie Night, for a fun and easy way for the whole family to learn about health.

Is anybody trying to change the food served in our schools? Chef Ann is! Check out her website and spread the word! I'm amazed at the blessing she is to so many children by cooking them healthier foods, http://www.chefannfoundation.org/.[140] Maybe you could be the next Chef Ann for your school district. Think about it!

Make extra food at dinner each night so there are lots of lunch packing choices. Fruits and veggies are great snacks, but pack something more filling like homemade muffins, pasta, beans and rice, potatoes, wraps, veggie sandwiches, burritos, and soups.

Yes, you can buy vegan food somewhere, but it's pretty hard to buy vegan food that's oil free and doesn't have nuts and dates and avocado and processed soy. Why don't you want all those things? They're delicious aren't they? And they're healthy fats too, aren't they? Here's the answer: It's too much fat. Most vegan diets are around 30% fat. That is the same fat content as the standard American diet. We really want to keep our fat intake under 10% to protect our heart. Most teenagers already have the beginning signs of heart disease and don't even know it. We don't want to eat things that have large amounts of fat in them. Your body only needs a very small amount of fat each day. If all you eat are starches, fruits and vegetables you will get all the fat your body needs. When you start adding fat to your diet, your body just stores it and disease begins to form.

There really is no cheaper food than plant based food, so you will be saving money by bringing your lunch on the road with you rather than stopping for lunch. Of course not only are you saving money but you are also saving your health, which is priceless.

Another "lunch love" for me are veggie sandwiches. Veggie wraps are great too, and you can even wrap your leftovers. Soups and stews and salad are delicious. What about the kids? Pack their lunches too. Pack veggie sandwiches or veggie wraps or bean burritos. I know what you're thinking, "but they love their school lunch," or "they get free school lunches," or "they won't eat what you pack them," or "I don't have time to pack them lunches," or you don't want to fight with them about it. As a mother of four children who went from a standard American diet to a low-fat whole food plant-based diet, I can assure you that it's not easy and they will complain for a while until they adjust to the new food. Lucky for me, as already mentioned, I only have one complainer out of the four. But it's still pretty brutal. We compromise. I do my best to parent with love. I'm trying to teach him to treat his body and our Earth well by making good food choices. I don't think force is the right way to parent, so this school lunch thing is giving me the opportunity to communicate and teach my kids. No one ever said parenting would be easy right?

More lunch ideas—how could I forget peanut butter and jelly sandwiches? I don't usually eat peanut butter and jelly sandwiches myself as I really try to avoid nuts, but I will pack them for the kids. The most nutritious PB&J is on 100% whole-grain bread, using peanut butter that's actually made of only peanuts and not full of oil and sugar, and jelly that's just fruit with minimal or no sweeteners. Fruit, muffins, veggies and homemade Larabars®. They are great snacks to go along with a packed lunch.

CHAPTER 44

MAKE YOUR OWN BIRTHDAY CAKES AND FROSTING

I KNOW IT's tempting to buy a cake, but it's really so easy to make one! Again, why eat all that white flour, white sugar, food color, eggs, oil and preservatives when you can make a cake with more wholesome ingredients? Or how about this, buy an organic mix with ingredients you can live with, and instead of adding oil and eggs add applesauce and egg replacer. I did that last night for my daughter's birthday party and enjoyed watching those cupcakes get devoured!

There are lots of options for the frosting too. Just google "vegan frosting" and try a few recipes; oil free is best. At our house we usually skip the frosting and top our cakes with a drizzle of honey, shredded coconut and some fresh fruit.

Or try this cake and frosting recipe:[141]

Beet Chocolate Cake

Ingredients

- *1 large beet*
- *water*
- *unsweetened apple sauce*
- *2 tbsp. water*
- *1 tsp. vanilla extract*
- *1 tsp. apple cider vinegar*
- *1 cup whole wheat flour (I like white whole wheat)*
- *1/2 cup unbleached white flour (or more whole wheat)*

- 1/2 cup cocoa
- 1 cup sugar
- 1 tbsp. cornstarch
- 2 tsp. baking soda
- 1/2 tsp. salt
- 1/4 tsp. cinnamon

Instructions
1. Peel and dice one large beet. Place the pieces in a saucepan with water to cover and boil until soft. (I've heard that you can buy canned beets, so you may want to skip this step–and the resulting red hands–by using pre-cooked beets.) Allow the beets to cool, and then drain them, reserving the red water for another purpose. Put the drained beets into the food processor with 1/4 cup (clear) water, and process until pureed.
2. Preheat the oven to 325 degrees. Oil or spray your cooking pan(s).
3. Put the pureed beets into a 2-cup measure. Add enough apple sauce to reach the 2-cup line. Add the 2 tablespoons water, vanilla extract, and apple cider to the beets and mix well.
4. Mix the dry ingredients together; then add the beet mixture and stir until well-combined. Bake for 35-60 minutes, depending on the size of pan you use: more for small, deep pans and less for a 9X13 pan. (I used a 9X13 pan, and it took 35 minutes.) Test by inserting a toothpick into the center; it's done when the toothpick comes out clean.
5. Allow to cool completely before cutting and serving.

Banana-Peanut Butter Sauce:

1/2 of a 12-ounce package lite, firm silken tofu
1 banana
2 tbsp. natural peanut butter
1/4-1/3 cup agave nectar, to taste
1/4 tsp. vanilla
1/2 tsp. lemon juice

Blend all ingredients in a food processor or blender until smooth. Refrigerate until needed. The sauce will thicken in the fridge, so it's best to give it time to chill if you plan to sandwich it between layers of cake. (Just for fun, the next time I make this, I'll add a couple of drops of the beet juice to it to give it a slightly pink color.) Serve over cake.

Preparation time: 20 minute(s) | Cooking time: 55 minute(s)

Number of servings (yield): 8

Nutrition Facts

1/8 of cake alone (no topping): 212 calories, 5% calories from fat, 1 gram fat, 471mg sodium, 209mg potassium 50g carbohydrates, 4.5g fiber, 4g protein.

Banana-Peanut Butter Sauce adds the following, per serving: 91 calories, 2.5 g fat, 63mg sodium, 115mg potassium, 13g carbohydrates, 1g fiber, 6g protein.

CHAPTER 45

LEARN ABOUT GRAINS

GRAINS ARE MEANT to be the staff of life, as we've learned from our ancestors' diets of grains and starches. We've also learned that a whole food, plant based diet prevents and reverses all modern diseases. We get confused and think meat is the staff of life.

I was really excited when I learned about grains as I knew I was eating too much meat. I didn't know what else to eat without gaining weight. In the Mormon health code[142] that I was trying to follow; it says to eat meat sparingly and only in times of winter or famine and it's pleasing to God if we do not eat them at all. Parts of this health code are mandatory for church members and parts are optional. The mandatory parts are no alcohol, tea, coffee and tobacco. The recommend but optional parts are to eat little to no meat and make grains your staff of life. Also eat foods in their season all with prudence and thanksgiving. Great blessing are promised for following this health code and the recommendations and promise goes out to the entire world and was announced in 1833!

Chef Brad's TV show called Fusion Grain Cooking is how I learned about cooking with grains. Then I started adding grains to recipes I already made. I also read his book, Cooking with Chef Brad, Those Wonderful Grains. You can also find all his cooking shows and recipes on his website www.ChefBrad.com.[143] Chef Brad is so much fun to watch, and he's so knowledgeable about cooking and grains! I do modify Chef Brad's recipes to make them plant based. I love what I've learned from Chef Brad about grains.

CHAPTER 46

DO WE NEED PORTION CONTROL?

Do you need portion control on a whole food, plant based diet? The answer is, NO! Portion Control is not needed. You can eat until you are full and satisfied and still lose weight, and be at your ideal weight and stay there. But ("and there's always the big butt," as Peewee Herman says, ha-ha :-)), if you are an emotional eater and you stuff yourself with food all day trying to soothe your soul, you probably won't be able to get to your ideal weight as fast. Stuffing yourself with whole food is much better for your health than stuffing yourself with the standard American diet, but why are you stuffing yourself?

In chapter 97 and 99 I talk more about getting to the bottom of overeating. I was finally able to overcome that in a quick and simple way with a method of subconscious belief change. I also describe how to do it the harder way because I know the easy way is not for everyone.

Now back to the portion sizes; if you are eating to eat, have at it! Whole food plant based food, that is. Remember that avocados and nuts are very high in fat and you should not be eating them, except for a bit of flavor or if you need to gain weight and if you have no heart disease, blood pressure or cholesterol issues. Dried fruit is also very high in calories, so eat it sparingly, unless you don't need to lose weight. You can eat an unlimited amount of potatoes, corn, rice, sweet potatoes, vegetables, beans, grains, legumes and fruits; and it would be nearly impossible to gain a pound if you are eating to eat and not constantly overeating for emotional pain control.

If you have weight to lose, eat 50% starches, 40% veggies and 10% fruit. You will shed about 10 pounds per month with this whole food, plant based plan. Remember, cut out the fats, including oils. Whole foods have all the fat you need. There's no need to put extra fat on your food and will slow down your weight loss. As Dr. McDougall says, "the fat you eat is the fat you wear."[144] You wear that fat on the inside and outside of your body, which damages your body image and also damages your 60,000 miles of veins and arteries. If you are not trying to lose weight and just want to be healthy, you can eat 80% starch if you like and you won't gain a pound. If you are coming off the high fat, empty calorie standard American diet, you will still lose weight even on large quantities of low fat starches like potatoes and rice.

When you eat starches, it takes your body about 30% of the calories you eat to convert the food to fuel your body. When you eat fat, there is almost no conversion, which is one reason why it's easier to store the extra calories on your body. Carbohydrates/starches have four calories per gram and fat has nine calories per gram. That being said, you can see that you can eat twice as many carbs as fats; and then when you add in the 30% conversion rate to turn those carbs into fuel, you can eat almost three times as much for the same calorie count. We are not counting calories on this diet, but I just wanted to explain why you can eat so much and not gain weight, and almost everyone loses weight eating a plant based diet. I have eaten more in this past year than I probably did in the past three years combined, yet my weight has dropped. Plus, I was more satisfied than ever, as my body was made to run on glucose which is what starches are made of. When you give your body the right fuel it functions as it was meant to.[145]

If you fill your stomach with starches, think how much fuller you will feel on less calories, compared to putting a small amount of calorie dense fat into your stomach that gives you little satiation. You'll just want more. Choose starches!

CHAPTER 47

DON'T HAVE A "CHEAT DAY"

IF YOU ARE trying to get off the SAD diet, don't pick times to cheat; that will only make it harder. Like an addict trying to quit a bad habit, scheduling a chance to cheat once in a while is not the way to kick the habit! This does not mean that you can never cheat, but don't plan on it. If you do cheat, be prepared, because you are most likely going to feel miserable. If you keep your plane full of jet fuel and then try to fly it on unleaded, it just doesn't work right and you wonder how you ever managed before on that unhealthy fuel! When you plan to cheat, and then you cheat when you don't plan to as well, before you know it you are cheating all the time and you keep that SAD taste alive. Let it go! It's hard, I know; it took me many years to get to this understanding, but I know that you can do it! It's so worth it to avoid disease and the misery that goes with it.

In his book *Prevent and Reverse Heart Disease*, Dr. Caldwell B. Esselstyn Jr., MD has a whole chapter called "Moderation Kills.[146]" He explains how there have been heart studies done that show that people who reduced their fat intake do not have less cancers, heart attacks etc. He says the problem with these reports is that even the low fat eaters are still eating three times the fat of a plant based diet. He compares this research to cars. If a car hits a stone wall at 90 miles per hour and all occupants die and then you repeat at 80 miles per hour and all occupants die and then repeat at 70 miles per hour, and all occupants die. Can you really say that speed does not matter in a car accident? What about 10 miles per hour? Would everyone die then? The same goes for diet. A country full of disease calls for drastic measures. Meatless Mondays are not sufficient to fight disease. We need to slow this ride to 10 miles per hour if we want to save our lives.

CHAPTER 48

GOT AILMENTS?

WHEN WE HAVE health challenges it's for a reason. Our bodies are reacting to a problem. We need to be grateful for our bodies warning system and listen. Do we have frequent aliments and not look for the cause? Most often, the cause of modern disease is our food. How could it not be? We fill our bodies full of it every single day. A perfect example is me and dairy. For my entire life I've been a gum chewer. I never liked the taste in my mouth, so I had mint gum in my mouth since I was about 12 years old. As I got healthy, I switched to natural gums, so I was not chewing on chemicals all day, even though they were more expensive, not as tasty, and the flavor didn't last as long. Chewing healthy gum was still better than that weird taste in my mouth. Fast forward to "no more dairy for me," and guess what? My mouth tastes fine; there is no more weird taste. So why was I not looking for the cause of my issue, why was I just covering it up? Where else was I doing that with messages my body was sending me. Sadly, "talk to the hand" was what I usually told my body when it was trying to alert me to something. I've learned better now.

Consider what you put in your mouth. It really does make a huge difference! If you've got a health problem, start eliminating foods and see if you can find the culprit. One problem is that some foods that are bad for us like meat, for example, might not cause you any immediate problems; but they can cause cancer growth inside your body. There are definitely certain foods to avoid. Animal products, oils and processed foods will cause disease. But some of us have sensitivities to other foods, so why keep feeding your body something that bothers you? Respect yourself, care for yourself, understand yourself and listen to yourself. Figure out what food is causing your issue and stop eating it. Be kind to yourself.

I've also found that our emotions can wreak havoc on our bodies as well as cause reaction and irritations to food. Most of the time we don't even put two and two together in that arena. To overcome these reactions and irritations, check out my www.BalancedYou.org page.[147] Let's all feel better!

CHAPTER 49

B12

THERE IS A lot of debate out there about vitamin B12 and whether there are any plant based foods that have B12. The best information I've read about B12 is that if you are vegan you need to supplement a bit. You can have your blood tested to see if you need B12, or get a muscle test, or just take some.

Dr. McDougall says, "The risk of a B12 deficiency disease is extremely small (1 in a million) and takes more than three years to develop. To avoid even small risks, take this supplement. The need is fewer than 5 micrograms (mcg) daily. However, the smallest doses sold in stores are 500 mcg. Likely, no side effects [will] occur from the excess. Once a week is adequate."[148]

Some say that this B12 issue proves that humans are meant to eat meat. And let's just say they are right. The problem in America is we don't eat meat; we devour it while we destroy our planet and our bodies by eating like carnivores every meal of every day. We consume 70 billion animals a year. This is not natural for our bodies, our earth, or the poor animals!

B12 is actually not a vitamin but a bacteria found in animals. If you don't eat animals, you don't get B12. B12 lives in our guts but needs to be higher in our intestinal tract to break down food. For most people, B12 lasts for many years in their bodies from the supply they have built up from eating animals.[149] However, it's better to be safe than sorry. When in doubt, take a B12 supplement.

CHAPTER 50

HUMAN CARNIVORY

I'M SAD TO say that in the past I really didn't worry too much about the Earth. I would say that I cared but I didn't show it through my actions. I didn't think little old me could make a whole lot of impact by changing my ways. I've learned that is quite the opposite of the truth.

Probably the first thing that hit me was the California drought, right here where I live. People get upset if you leave the water running while you brush your teeth, but they don't care that it takes 1,800 to 4,200 gallons of water to produce one pound of beef versus 34 gallons of water to produce one pound of potatoes. There are lighted signs on our freeways that say "limit outdoor watering," yet no one says to limit meat consumption. When I stopped buying meat for my family of six, and we were huge meat eaters, how much water did our house save? Multiply that by all those we've shared this message with, and who they've shared it with, and we really can make a difference!

As I've learned more about the Earth and the devastation we are causing by consuming so much meat, I've found it very interesting that what's good for us is also good for the Earth.

I listened to a lecture[150] by William Ripple, PhD., an ecologist for 30 years at Oregon State University. He explained the effects of human carnivory. It's very complex and affects us in many ways. The problem is, we do not see the bad effects of our diet on our Earth immediately, just as we don't see the bad effects inside our bodies immediately. We hear about global warming, and we hear about species dying off, greenhouse gases, trouble in our oceans, deforestation etc.; but if you go outside it still looks pretty fine out there. We still have water and air, wildlife and beautiful places to explore. However, when you look into the details of what we are doing to our Earth, it's like getting the wind knocked out of you.

Again, this can be likened to our diets. We eat a burger and nothing catastrophic happens, right? Maybe not to our untrained eye, but there are definite effects happening inside your body. As Dr. Esselstyn says, "Every segment of our bodies is comprised of cells, and every individual cell is protected by an outer coat. This cell membrane is almost unimaginably delicate-just one hundred-thousandth of a millimeter thick. Yet it is absolutely essential to the integrity and healthy function of the cell. And it is extremely vulnerable to injury. Every mouthful of oils and animal products, including dairy foods, initiates an assault on these membranes and, therefore, on the cells they protect."[151]" Then we cause this same damage over, and over, and over again. Our bodies can't recover, and start to become diseased. When we eat in a way that our bodies were not meant to eat, and we farm/fish/destroy the Earth to produce the animal products we want, there is a price to pay. Do you know anyone with a modern disease? Diseases like cancer, heart disease, diabetes, obesity, high blood pressure and high cholesterol to name a few. These are very real, and are the effect of what we put in our mouths each day.

The Earth was designed in a masterful way. All species have a place and a purpose. When species are killed off due to human carnivory, there is a price to be paid. Again, we can make a difference. Look at basketball star Yao Ming. Ming refuses to eat shark fin soup. Since he started this campaign, shark killing is down by 50%.[152] How awesome is that?

How does human carnivory kill off species, you ask? It's because the livestock take the land and the resources, and then leave the land barren. It's not just the livestock that are involved, of course; it's the people and our greed and demands to have what we want when we want it. We need to take a step back and look at the ramifications of our choices and stop the destruction now, before it's too late for our bodies and our Earth.

CHAPTER 51

FAMILY MOVIE NIGHT

ONE OF THE best ways to get your family on board with healthy eating is to educate them. But do they really want to listen to a lecture from mom? Mine didn't, so I did the sneaky thing, turned on a movie in the family room. Before I knew it, I was surrounded by my family wanting to see what mom was watching. These movies below had a huge impact on them and me.

My favorite health movie is *Forks Over Knives,* **(https://www.youtube.com/watch?v=DZb-35oV_7E).**[153] *Forks Over Knives* shows the benefits of a plant-based diet on your health and disease reversal.

The next movie is the *Widowmaker* **(http://widowmakerthemovie.com/).**[154] 700,000 Americans die from heart disease each year; one third of them don't know they have heart disease until they have a heart attack and die. There is a method to find heart problems before it's too late. It is cheap, easy, and simple, but it's being covered up by some people in the medical industry. Of course you could just eat plants and prevent and reverse heart disease instead of scanning your body to see what damage you've done.

Cowspiracy **(http://www.cowspiracy.com/)**[155] is another great movie. It explains how the real destruction of our environment is the raising and killing of 70 billion animals per year for our consumption, and no one will talk about it. Not even the environmentalist groups! Why not?

PlantPureNation **(https://www.youtube.com/watch?v=9E6sa0OtjSE)**[156] is another favorite. I actually broke down sobbing from watching this movie! My husband called at the height of my break down to say "hi." My kids were holding my hands and rubbing my head while I tried to speak to my husband. I cried something like this into the phone with my kids watching me. "It's just wrong that so many people are suffering from diseases that could be cured with a plant-based diet, but they don't know about it because their doctors are not trained in nutrition! Lobbyists, government, and Big Business lie to fatten their wallets, and people are suffering needlessly. I need to tell everyone how to find health and cure disease!" My husband tried to console me and let me know that I am doing the right thing by sharing this message with others.

My ugly crying did calm down after a bit but I really do get worked up over this topic. I think that everyone should know what they are doing to themselves and the Earth. Then they can make an informed choice. The opposite is going on today. We are told that meat, dairy, eggs and oils give us health. It's a flat-out money making lie!

In *PlantPure Nation*, Nelson Campbell, the son of T. Colin Campbell, with a Ph.D. in Nutritional Science and co-author of *The China Study*, tries to get Congress to pass a law telling people the truth about what foods hurt them and cause disease and which foods bring good health. Even with tons of scientific evidence to support plant based eating for the past 100 years, not many lawmakers will listen to the truth. There are 100,000 people in the U.S. with type 2 diabetes and they could all be cured in the next 10 days on a plant based diet if they had the information and, of course, chose to follow it. My trouble is not with those that choose not to follow; my heart aches for those that don't know the truth and suffer needlessly. I am flabbergasted at the power of large companies to hide and distort the truth. I can't fathom a company causing people to suffer just to line its pockets, and it happens in America all day, every day. Not just with diabetes, but with all chronic diseases in America. If we put the right fuel in our body, it works perfectly. If we put lawn mower fuel in our jet engine, it starts to sputter with cancer, heart disease, diabetes, Alzheimer's, Parkinson's, dementia, obesity, MS, stroke, kidney failure, pneumonia, blood infections, liver disease, and high blood pressure, just to name a few of the problems. We can prevent this.

Have you ever tried to grow a garden? It's fun, rewarding, healthful, delicious and organic but wow, it's hard work. Learn the secret to growing a garden without even tilling or watering! I can't wait to plant my Back to Eden garden! **(https://vimeo.com/28055108)**[157]

CHAPTER 52

KINDNESS BEGINS WITH ME

FROM A LITTLE church jingle I learned as a child, "I want to be kind to everyone (including animals!), for that is right, you see. So I say to myself, remember this, kindness begins with me."

Seventy billion animals are raised to be slaughtered for food every year, and that does not include what we are doing to our oceans. I don't think I need to go into the horror stories of those poor animals' living conditions or lives as most of us have seen documentaries showing what's really going on. Think about this question. Would you eat differently if you had to raise and kill the animals yourself that you wanted to eat? I think it's out of sight, out of mind, with our eating choices nowadays. Most of us don't think that an animal had to die for us to enjoy our dinner; we just eat our meat and that's that. We also don't think of the suffering animals endured while being raised, or the resources of our Earth that were used up to produce them.

I remember back to the days when I didn't eat a plant based diet and I was heating some chicken nuggets for my son. I put the chicken nuggets and barbecue sauce in front of him and said, "eat your chicken, it's good for you. You need your protein so you can grow big and strong and healthy." Yes, I too was sold on the American diet lies! My little son looked at me with a confused and concerned look in his eye. In a soft and shaky voice he said, "You mean chicken is chicken?" He was blown away. He wandered around the house all day with a glazed look on his face, whispering "chicken is chicken." I thought it was so funny at the time but now I can see he was sincerely concerned about the animals I was feeding him. Did he ask for an animal to be killed and fed to him? No! Maybe we should be more like my son and realize what we are doing.[158] The last time I cooked meat for my family, I reached into the freezer to grab that last package of ground turkey that I had purchased and I felt really guilty because my kitchen and pantry were full of food and yet I wanted to eat an animal instead. My food choices that night required killing a living creature, using up exorbitant amounts of our Earth's resources, and damaging my body— just because it was habit, we liked the taste, and we used to think it was good for us. I decided that night to never cook meat again, unless it was a matter of famine or hunger and we didn't have any other food choices.

CHAPTER 53

DON'T DO EVERYTHING THE DOCTOR TELLS YOU

My husband came home from the doctor's office the other day and told me that the doctor said for him to drink more cows' milk instead of almond milk and to eat more animal protein. The problem with doctors telling you how to eat is that most of them don't study nutrition. Doctors hear the same diet propaganda that we do. This propaganda comes from the companies that are trying to sell us their products. They spend hundreds of millions of dollars per year to convince us that their food is the best and even the healthiest. Maybe it's the coolest food too (cue a famous person sporting a milk mustache). Sometimes, as ALWAYS, it's better to study a product from the scientific data, not the magazine ads. I'm not saying that all doctors are alike regarding nutrition but it's not their area of expertise or study. You don't ask your plumber about your electrical problems, so don't ask your medical doctor about nutrition. It's just not what doctors are trained to know.

I was very excited to learn about Dr. Scott Stoll, during a February 2016 McDougall Advanced Study weekend. Dr. Stoll is teaching doctors about nutrition and teaching them how to prescribe whole foods instead of drugs and surgery. Dr. Stoll found that his patients were all sick and tired, and the only method he found that could cure them was nutrition. The best part is, it's cheap and easy and anyone can do it. Eating healthy is not for the rich or the elite, it's for everyone.

Check out Dr. Stoll's Plantrician Project Mission and go to his website, http://plantricianproject.org/plant-based-docs to find a plant based doctor near you. "The Plantrician Project Mission: To educate, equip and empower our physicians and healthcare practitioners with knowledge about the indisputable benefits of plant-based nutrition. To provide them with the resources they, in turn, use to inform and inspire their patients to shift from the Western industrialized diet to a life-changing, whole-food, plant-based way of living.[159]"

CHAPTER 54

SWITCH YOUR SYRUP

GUESS WHAT? YOU'RE Buying Fake Maple Syrup![160]

Last summer, my husband, daughter and I were staying at a mountain cabin we share with other family members. We took some time to clean out the refrigerator and pantry .Nothing was rotten, just tossing things that had expired, dressings that were mostly empty, etc. You know those mystery mustards, oils, random canned items. I even found boxes of lime jello that expired in 2004 (I would have tossed those expired or not!)

In the back of the refrigerator, I found 2 mostly empty bottles of Log Cabin syrup. It was expired, but I was going to toss it anyway. It has been years since I have bought that stuff, so I took a moment to read the ingredient label. YIKES!

It got me to thinking how many people aren't really aware that most of these syrups that are sold at the store are NOT maple syrup at all! It is shocking to me because nowhere on the label do these products say 'maple syrup' but most consumers do not know the difference.

They aren't real maple syrup folks! They are a combo of high fructose corn syrup, fake colors and artificial flavors essentially poison, in my opinion!

We all know, somewhere in the back of our brains, that maple syrup comes from maple sap from maple trees. In my mind, I have images of some frosty morning, gathering the sap and making the Syrup.

According to World's Healthiest Foods, "the sap is clear and almost tasteless and very low in sugar content when it is first tapped. It is then boiled to evaporate the water producing syrup with the characteristic flavor and color of maple syrup and sugar content of 60%."

Unfortunately, Big Food has taken over and even a simple, delicious treat as maple syrup has been corrupted and most of the syrups today are totally fake!

This is yet another reason why reading ingredient labels are THE MOST IMPORTANT thing you can do on your real food journey!

If you start to look closely at your grocery aisle, you will see many of the brands are called 'syrup' or 'table syrup' or 'maple-flavored syrup'. This is because only 100% pure maple syrup can be called 'maple syrup'.

When we first made the switch to 100% pure, organic maple syrup our son revolted and swore he'd never eat pancakes or waffles or French toast again! After about six months he gave in one hungry morning and tried it. He looked at me, amazed about how good the formerly "gross" syrup tasted. After that, it was all I could do to keep maple syrup on the shelf before we ran out of it. A few months later, my husband took the kids out to breakfast one morning. I loved the stories my son told when they got home about the sticky, disgusting restaurant syrup. Ha!

Maple syrup is also a delicious sweetener that you can use in cooking and baking. Yum! It's typically the only sweetener I use.

Tip: if there is a Costco near you, the 100% pure organic maple syrup is about half the price there compared to health food stores.

CHAPTER 55

TORTILLA CHIPS AND SALSA

MAKING TORTILLA CHIPS and salsa is fun, easy and healthy. Get some non-GMO, no lard or oil corn tortillas and turn the oven on to high broil. Place the tortillas on top of each other in stacks of three or four, and using good kitchen scissors, cut them into eighths. Lay the triangles on a cookie sheet and sprinkle with a bit of ink Himalayan salt on them, if you like. Place the triangles in the oven for three to six minutes, checking every minute or you'll be testing your smoke alarm! Once they are a nice, light golden brown, pull them out, flip them over and repeat; but the back side cooks faster, so don't forget that timer every minute until you know how long it takes in your oven!

For the salsa put some ripe tomatoes, onions, cilantro, garlic and jalapeño if you like it hot. Puree and serve. Delicious!

What else are you buying that you could make in your kitchen? When you make and or grow your own food, it's usually cheaper, healthier, fresher and tastier!

If you'd like to watch a video of the GreenSmoothieGirl[161] making chips and salsa check out this video, https://www.youtube.com/watch?v=qJnlgoomU5M. I'd recommend you skip the spraying the cookie sheet with oil step however. Ole!

CHAPTER 56

THE CARBOHYDRATE MYTH

SHOULD YOU AVOID whole carbs like potatoes, pasta, grains, corn, and rice? NO! Should you avoid processed carbs like pastries, chips, crackers, anything boxed or bagged? YES! Whole food carbs are wonderful and provide nutrients, energy, protein and carbohydrates. They provide your body with all the phytonutrients it needs to function at its best. If your body was at its best, what would be different? Your body wants to get there. You should let it!

Carbs are so satisfying! It's easy for me to understand and believe that carbohydrates are what our bodies are made to eat. I've learned that to be true from my study of health, plus reading a study of the past 15,000-plus years about the world's population eating grains and starches (like potatoes, rice and wheat) as their staple for health and survival.[162] Now, as I feed my body those same foods that it was designed to eat, and listen to the response, my body is satisfied. Our bodies want to eat grains and other starches; and when we do so, we feel satiated and satisfied.

Today, for lunch, I had a plate of whole grain pasta with an oil free and sugar free marinara sauce, green peas, green salad with fig vinegar for dressing, and a slice of warm whole grain bread. That one slice of bread turned to two before my delicious plate was done, because I ran out of bread before I ran out of spaghetti and we can't have that! The pasta was steaming hot and the tomato sauce was the best, just tomatoes and spices, no added oils, etc. When I finished my meal I felt so satisfied. My stomach was full and my brain was happy. Food is designed to fill your stomach, which will satisfy and nourish and strengthen your body. Your brain runs on sugar; not white table sugar (preferably), but glucose. We, as humans, have a high amount of amylase in our saliva. Amylase is an enzyme that breaks down starches and converts them to glucose, fueling our body and brain.[163] My brain was happy after I ate. When my blood sugar rose and my stomach filled, my body knows it's full and satisfied and can stop searching for nutrition and satisfaction.

I just ate a healthy meal full of carbs, protein, phytonutrients, vitamins and minerals. The great part, besides the taste, was that the meal was large yet low in calories. My stomach is full and my body will use the calories, not store them. But even better than that, there were no animal products or oils or chemicals that will cause disease in my body. And when I was finished, I was not searching for chocolate as I used to when I'd eaten salads and meat for lunch. I don't need or want anything else when I give my body the right fuel.

Why don't Americans eat more carbs? Everyone knows that if you want to lose weight you reduce eating the carbs, right? Actually, that is one way to lose weight because it actually makes your body sick and throws it into survival mode, trying to function without glucose. A much healthier way is to feed your body carbohydrates and not the animal products, oils and chemicals. By using this plan, you will lose weight and add health, not lose weight and add disease.

I have never eaten more carbohydrates than I do now. I've never been healthier, judging by how I feel, and I have great blood work too. I've never weighed less and I don't have to fight to keep my weight low, as I used to do every day of my life from about 10 years old to age 39, when I found this diet. I just stay at my ideal weight eating as much as I want, whenever I want. I eat grains and other starches like potatoes, fruits and vegetables. Don't believe the rumors. Say YES to carbs! Eat the least processed whole grain carbs possible with no added fats or chemicals. Here's to your health, satisfaction and success!

CHAPTER 57

NO MORE BROKEN HEARTS

How low can you go? How low can you go? How low can you go on animal product consumption?

Those are the questions from Dr. Robert Ostfeld, M.D., M.Sc., Director of Preventative Cardiology and Associate Professor of Clinical Medicine at Montefiore Medical Center[164], in a 2016 McDougall Advanced Study Weekend. Dr. Ostfeld said that he was frustrated that he could help his patients a little with medications and surgeries, but not enough to feel that he was doing all he could. Dr. Ostfeld was searching for answers and read *The China Study*, and immediately he added the plant based diet to his client recommendations. Not only was it good for their hearts, but also for every major system in their bodies and for the planet too. Dr. Ostfeld said he literally had patients who cried as they told him how much better they felt on a plant based diet. These patients got their lives back.

Dr. Ostfeld says that 65% of 12-14-year-olds in the U.S. have early signs of cholesterol disease that is already damaging their blood vessels. No wonder there are two heart attacks every minute in the United States. Heart disease is the number one killer of men and women. We know how prevalent breast cancer is, but the incidence of heart disease is seven times higher for women than breast cancer is. It's "normal" to die from heart disease in the U.S. The sad thing is that modern diseases are preventable, and many are reversible, with a plant based diet.

To prevent and reverse disease, do the animal product limbo! The lower you go on animal product consumption, the healthier you are. This has been proved, over and over and over again. If just believe what you hear, you think you need animal protein when it's actually the protein that is causing the disease. Don't be duped by companies selling you their products! Don't be fooled by your body that thinks it needs your current favorite foods. You'd be amazed about how much you can change if your health is important to you. You've can do this!

Why do we get so confused about what's good for us? Take the example of advertising dollars spent in the Super Bowl in 2004. Eight fast food chains spent $2.3 billion on their ads compared to federal spending for the "five a day program," which had a $4.9 million dollar budget. If you convert those dollar amounts to time that's 73 years versus two months. No wonder we think it's okay to eat burgers!

Did you see in the New York Times[165] that the president of the American College of Cardiology, Kim Williams, MD recommended a plant based diet on August 6th, 2014? The word is slowly getting out!

I'm so glad. There is so much unneeded suffering. This information is not new. It's been discussed in scientific studies for over 100 years! There was a headline in the New York Times on September 24th, 1907 (that year is not an error) that says Cancer Increases Among Meat Eaters. And there were many, many studies to prove it, even back then.

Read *The China Study* if you want to see the proof that animal products will give you disease. I had become a bit confused, thinking that it was the fat and the cholesterol in the animal protein that was causing disease, but Dr. T. Colin Campbell, author of *The China Study* recently reminded me in a webcast that it's actually the animal protein itself that causes disease. It does not matter if it's chicken, fish, milk or red meat.

Dr. Ostfeld says that scientist have discovered a new gene in carnivores called Neu5GC that people don't have. They believe this might be the reason that people get cancer from meat.

Did you know that you have 60,000 miles of blood vessels in your body?!? The Earth's circumference is 25,000 miles, to put that in perspective. That's a lot of pipes to keep clean! Americans are doing the opposite by clogging their arteries in their youth, which is why this is the first generation that will live shorter life spans than their parents. Some people say, "I'm going to die anyway, why not enjoy myself?" Look at any cancer patient. Where is their joy? Look at any family who lost a parent or grandparent to a heart attack. Where is their joy? Look at any modern disease. There is nothing pleasurable about it.

Please don't forget, a plant based diet includes mashed potatoes and gravy. We are not talking about living on greens!

CHAPTER 58

SNACK ON!

KEEP HEALTHY SNACKS in your car. How many times does "Mom's taxi service" run longer than you expected, or you pick up a car load of famished kids? I ALWAYS keep healthy snacks in my car to ward off hunger for myself and my children.

If at all possible, before you leave bag up some sliced fruits and veggies for easy snacking. A loaf of bread or homemade muffins are wonderfully filling if they need more than fruit and veggies.

I try to always have healthy options sitting out for my kids to grab such as slicked cantaloupe or grapes. Cereal is a great snack with homemade nut milk. Look for a whole grain cereal that does not have oil in it.

If it's just me in the car, and now that my kids are getting older that actually happens, I love apples. Apples are one of my all-time favorite snacks. It's very common for me to bring an apple in my car, because I seem to get the munchies when I'm out running around and an apple in my car can take the heat and is ready and waiting for me when I want it.

The thing that you don't want to snack on that used to always be my favorite snack, and probably one of the reasons why I was always trying to lose weight, is nuts. Nuts are packed with fat and calories. While a couple might be good for you, who eats a couple of nuts and stops there? Nuts don't raise your blood sugar enough, and they don't fill your stomach enough to find satisfaction quickly. By the time you've stopped eating them, you have a huge overabundance of fat and calories and possibly sodium too if they are salted nuts. For better heart health and better body shape, snack on starches (carbohydrates), fruits and veggies.

Check out 25 Oil- Free Vegan Savory Snacks here, http://plantbaseddietitian.com/25-oil-free-vegan-savory-snacks/. Delish!

CHAPTER 59

SHOULD YOU BE GLUTEN FREE?

SHOULD YOU BE eating gluten free? You hear it everywhere you go, but why? It's a buzzword and a special diet that people follow, and they don't even understand why. There are also untrue books out there like Grain Brain and Wheat Belly that make you think that gluten is bad for the general population, but when you look at the research on who was tested, the studies were run on people with gluten intolerance and celiac disease, according to Dr. John McDougall.[166]

The simple answer is no! You should not be eating gluten free UNLESS you have a health issue with gluten. It's true that people are more sensitive to gluten nowadays because of the GMOs and the pesticides; but when people don't eat gluten, and gluten doesn't bother them but they think they should avoid it, what do these gluten-free people turn to? Most of them turned to more processed gluten free grains or animal products, which are far, far worse, causing cancer, diabetes and heart disease. So don't look for gluten free; look for animal product free and oil free and 100% whole grain. No more gluten confusion.

CHAPTER 60

CASHEW CHEESE, COCONUT YOGURT-YUM, BUT

REMEMBER, PLANT BASED whole food is our nutrition goal. We want natural foods, not processed foods. Sometimes when we are eating healthy, we try to replace one food with another look-alike that is typically another processed food. Regarding dairy, the look-alikes in the store have too much fat, and some nut cheeses still have the milk protein casein in it. It may be lactose free, but casein is what Dr. T. Colin Campbell used in his trials to turn cancer on and off. We don't want any of that in our bodies.

If your family can't live without cheese, make it. It's not very hard to do and there are a lot of great nut cheese recipes. Just remember, if you're trying to lose weight, you don't want to be eating cheese. Even homemade nut cheese.

I make a cashew cheese spread, see my recipe section under the Sides, Sauces, and More, that I put on garlic bread when we have spaghetti, and my kids also like to put in on their toast or bagels. I also put it on pizza and in enchiladas. The ingredients are very easy and it has a great shelf life in the fridge once it's made.

What about yogurt? Contrary to popular belief and advertising, it's not good for you. It's full of casein, the animal protein that turns on cancer, and sugar, which feeds cancer growth. This is a scary and terrible combination! Isn't it amazing that companies can market yogurt as healthy because they put some healthy bacteria in it, and tell you it's full of the protein your body needs? Your body does need protein from whole foods to make it strong and healthy, but not animal protein that causes disease. Do you see how the truth gets twisted for profits?

Are there alternatives? Yes, coconut yogurt is delicious. But high fat and high sugar and is not what I would call a whole food. Try putting fruit on oatmeal instead of yogurt. Your heart will say "thank you."

In plain and simple terms, the cause of obesity is:[167]

1. *Eating too much of foods that are too concentrated in calories. Especially the fats and oils which are present in natural foods or are added to foods being prepared for the table. "The fat you eat is the fat you wear."*
2. *Not eating enough starches, because of the mistaken notion that "starches make you fat." The carbohydrate in starches satisfies the hunger drive. Fat offers very little satisfaction for the hunger drive.*
3. *Not enough exercise.*

Switch to foods that provide fewer calories and more fibers. A change to a diet of starches, vegetables, and fruits will allow you to eat twice as much, as measured by volume, and yet take in only half as many calories as you did while stuffing yourself with the dishes offered by the rich American diet. As an added bonus, you're eating helpful, healthful foods that contain no cholesterol and no additives, lots of fibers and clean-burning carbohydrates, and moreover, all low in fats and in sodium content.

A quick recap: all dairy replacements are better than dairy for your health; BUT, if you are trying to lose weight, nothing will work faster than cutting the fat out of your diet. If you don't want to lose weight, make your own dairy replacements and enjoy them.

CHAPTER 61

NUTRITIONAL YEAST

It's interesting how your tastes change as you switch from the standard American diet to a whole food, plant based diet. I never thought that I could eat Italian food without Parmesan cheese, or Mexican food without sour cream and diary cheese, but now those things taste bad to me and I can't imagine eating them.

When I first tasted nutritional yeast I wasn't a fan of it. If I couldn't have Parmesan cheese on my spaghetti I would rather eat it plain. But as time went on, the taste of nutritional yeast grew on me and now I love it and use it to flavor sauces, dips, spreads and cheeses.

I love Susan's article on her blog, The Fat Free Vegan. *"What the Heck is Nutritional Yeast?*[168]*" Of all the ingredients I use in my recipes, the one I'm asked about the most is nutritional yeast. I've been cooking with it for so long that I forget how strange it must sound to people who are new to vegan cooking. Neither the word "nutritional" nor the word "yeast" conjures up mouthwatering images; but the truth is, it's one of the few health food store ingredients that I wouldn't want to have to do without, not because of its nutritional value, but because of its flavor. So what is it, why should you use it, and where can you find it?*

What It Is?

Nutritional yeast is made from a single-celled organism, Saccharomyces Cerevisiae, which is grown on molasses and then harvested, washed, and dried with heat to kill or deactivate it. Because it's inactive, it doesn't froth or grow like baking yeast does so it has no leavening ability. Don't worry; no animals are harmed in this process because yeasts are members of the fungi family, like mushrooms, not animals.

Nutritional yeast has such an unappealing name that somebody started calling it "nooch," and the name caught on in some corners of the Internet. The brand that most vegans use is Red Star Vegetarian Support Formula, because it is a good source of vitamin B12 and contains no whey, an animal product that is used in some other brands. In the U.K., nutritional yeast is sold under the Engevita brand, and in Australia as savory yeast flakes.

What It Isn't

Nutritional yeast is not the same as brewer's yeast, which is an ingredient used in the beer-making process and is very bitter. It's also not Torula yeast, which is grown on paper mill waste and is also not very tasty. And please do not try to substitute active dry yeast or baking yeast, which taste bad and will probably make a huge, frothy mess because they are alive.

Where Can I Find It?

You probably won't be able to find nutritional yeast in a typical grocery store. I buy it from the bulk bins at the local natural food store, where it is labeled "Vegetarian Support Formula." Larger grocery stores might have the Bob's Red Mill brand in the natural food section. If you can't find it locally, Amazon has several brands, including Red Star. Some brands of nutritional yeast taste better than others; so if you can, buy a little and taste it first, and if you don't like it, try another brand.

I use the flaked version of nutritional yeast, but it's also available in a powder. If you're using the powder, you will need only about half as much as the flakes.

Why Use It?

As you can guess from its name, nutritional yeast is packed with nutrition, particularly B vitamins, folic acid, selenium, zinc, and protein. It's low in fat, is gluten-free (check specific brands for certification), and contains no added sugars or preservatives. Because vitamin B12 is absent from plant foods unless it's added as a supplement, nutritional yeast that contains B12, such as Red Star Vegetarian Support Formula, is a great addition to the vegan diet (though

I strongly recommend taking a supplement as the only way to be sure you're getting enough). Not all nooch has B12, so check the label carefully before buying.

The vitamins and minerals are all well and good, but truthfully, I use nutritional yeast for its flavor, which has been described as cheesy, nutty, savory, and umami. Just a tablespoon or two can add richness to soups, gravies, and other dishes, and larger amounts can make "cheese" sauces and egg free scrambles taste cheesy and eggy.

Adding a small amount of nutritional yeast to a dish enhances the flavors present and helps to form a rich flavor base. If for some reason you can't find nutritional yeast, or can't use it, you can safely leave it out of recipes where it's used in small amounts as only a flavor enhancer; in some cases, miso or soy sauce can be used in a 1:3 ratio (1/3 of the amount of nooch called for), although both add sodium, so you may need to reduce the salt. In recipes where nutritional yeast provides the bulk of the flavor, such as vegan cheese sauces, it's best not to attempt to substitute it.

Nutritional yeast on popcorn: Does it contain MSG?

No. The savory, umami taste of nutritional yeast comes from glutamaic acid, an amino acid that is formed during the drying process. Glutamic acid is a naturally occurring amino acid found in many fruits and vegetables and is not the same as the commercial additive monosodium glutamate.

How do I use it?

If you're new to nutritional yeast, it's better to try it a little at a time rather than to dive right into a recipe that uses a lot of it. Try some of the suggestions below, using just a little until you develop a taste for it:

 Sprinkle it on popcorn.
 Stir it into mashed potatoes.
 Add a little to the cooking water for cheesy grits or polenta.
 Sprinkle nutritional yeast on any pasta dish.
 Make almond "Parmesan" by blending nutritional yeast with raw almonds in a food processor.
 Add a tablespoon or two to bean dishes to enhance the flavors.

Some have *concern that high amounts of synthetic folic acid may increase the risk of breast cancer. Most brands of nutritional yeast do contain added folic acid in varying amounts. If you are concerned about this, read the labels carefully and choose brands that contain as little as possible. I know of three brands of nutritional yeast that don't contain synthetic folic acid: Sari Foods, KAL Unfortified Yeast Flakes, and Dr. Fuhrman's Nutritional Yeast.*

One little tip from me, the gluten free nutritional yeast does not taste as good as the standard type. Get the regular nutritional yeast, not gluten free, if you can.

CHAPTER 62

MAKE YOUR OWN FLOUR

DO YOU KNOW how easy it is to make flour? I should say that it's easier than you think IF you have an electric mill and not a hand grinder. I had a hand grinder to start with, and I saw this awesome cornbread recipe made with popcorn kernels. I attached the hand crank to the kitchen table and begged the family to help me grind the popcorn. It took about a week of grinding until we had enough flour to make a batch of cornbread, and the kids said they would never touch that hand grinder again. I was able to get an electric grain mill, which surprisingly wasn't that expensive when compared with some other kitchen gadgets. To use a grain mill, just pour the grains in the top, turn it on, and about three minutes later you have more flour than you know what to do with.

It definitely saves money if you make your own flour, and you can make a variety of different combinations of flours that you can't buy in the store. Also, you know it's 100% whole grain because you're put the whole grains in the mill yourself. Buy organic grain if you can, so you're not eating pesticides along with your bread.

I learned to combine brown rice, spelt and barley from Chef Brad. He calls it "WonderFlour.[169]" It's a really great mix for all kinds of baking. Make sure that you add plenty of baking powder when using it or all your baking will come out dense and flat. I always seem to forget the baking powder on my first griddle full of pancakes, but I'm reminded quickly after wondering why my pancakes are so flat. Maybe I should look at my own recipes!

Back to the grains: if you store grains, it's really nice to know what to do with grains and how to eat them every day instead of looking at them in an emergency and not knowing what to do to them to feed them to your family. It's also great to know that you don't need and should not use eggs or oil in your bread. Use Ener-G egg replacer and skip the oil. My tummy is growling just from thinking about fresh baked bread!

CHAPTER 63

THEY WILL EAT WHAT YOU FEED THEM ... EVENTUALLY!

ONE OF MY daughters kindly reminded me the other night that she only eats what I feed her and what I buy her. It's so true. I had been slacking off a little on always having a plethora of fresh chopped veggies, fruit etc. because we are selling our house; and frankly, I was worn out from trying to keep the whole house and especially the kitchen spotless. They were snacking on cereal instead of fruits and veggies because I was tired! Her gentle reminder gave me the motivation I needed to start turning out those fruit and veggie trays between meals for them.

Keep the junk food out of the house. If there's no junk for them to eat, they don't eat junk. That doesn't mean that my kids never cheat on the plant based diet when they're away from home or beg dad to take them out to eat; but when they eat here, which is most of the time, they are eating wholesome foods. Some of my kids enjoy cheating on the plant based diet more than others. I have noticed, however, that the more anyone cheats, the harder it is to eat right. You get that taste for chemically enhanced, rich and fatty food. Then when you eat something pure and natural your taste buds want more simulation. Your taste buds will be happy with pure and natural food if you don't keep teasing them with the fat, salt, sugar and preservatives of the standard American diet.

I used to keep a stash of chocolate in my desk drawer, and my teenage daughters knew it and would come begging for some. Nowadays, I eat frozen grapes if I want a treat or dates or fruit.

Some of my kids graciously thank me for all my healthy cooking and tell me how delicious it is. With others it takes much more effort, skill, understanding and patience.

10 Tips From A Pediatrician: How To Feed Your Plant-Based Family Without Losing Your Mind[170]

1. Be a role model!
If your toddler sees you slurping down a juicy mango or eating crisp snap peas with delight, it's going to look much more appealing. In short, walk the talk. Those little creatures are smart, and they'll figure it out if you're not authentic.

2. Offer a variety (but not too many!) of great choices.
Provide two to three choices without placing any attachment to either choice. Apples or banana for snack? Let them have a say, but set them up for success.

3. Don't be a short-order cook.
I've made this mistake myself, so I say this with much personal experience. Make one meal for the whole family, with small accommodations as needed (i.e., spice level, food allergies, size of bites, etc.). If you start out making something different for everyone at the table, this will become your reality on a daily basis. And that's just exhausting.

4. Be patient and calm when introducing new foods.
Remember it can take upwards of ten times for a child to enjoy a new food. Try to keep the mood pleasant and certainly avoid getting into food battles. If you have school-aged children or adolescents who have firm preferences (and dislikes!), it can be a bit more challenging.

5. Invite instead of impose.
Nobody likes to be told what to do. If you've made some personal changes and are excited to share them with your family, don't be surprised if not everyone jumps on board right away. The first step may simply be to have a large salad at every meal, making sure to include foods that you know will be greeted with joy.

6. Don't be sneaky.
In addition to being told what to do, nobody likes to be tricked. The few leaves of hearty kale you covertly mixed into their morning smoothing could backfire. If

little ones detect bitterness or a less sweet version of their favorite smoothie, they will learn to distrust your offerings. A different approach could be: "I've added a secret ingredient, and I'm wondering if you can figure out what is?" or allow them to throw in as many leaves of spinach that they'd like and gradually work your way up.

7. Make it fun and creative.
Turning anything into a "bar" (i.e., salad, taco, rice bowls, etc.) is great way to get kids to try new ingredients or combinations. It also gives them some control over the meal by allowing them to add which and how much of each ingredient.

Although it sounds cliché, I find that when kids are actively involved with the food (from menu planning and shopping to chopping and simmering), they feel more invested and a part of the whole process. A quick example that comes to mind is our family's search for the perfect pesto. Many store-bought pestos contain dairy and my son is allergic to tree nuts. So, he decided he would search for a nut-free pesto recipe. We made a few small changes and together created a spinach-basil pesto that has become a family favorite. Don't feel pressured to have them involved with every meal. I like to think of it as an open door policy—they are welcome anytime! Sometimes it's as involved as helping to cook an entire meal and other times it's just wanting to have the fun of sautéing some onions or giving a quick stir to a soup.

8. Be a good listener.
If your child really dislikes something, be willing to hear them out and offer a reasonable substitute. I'm not talking about being a short-order cook (see above!), but if there is something you can do that makes the meal more enjoyable, go for it! One of my kids really dislikes warm or sautéed snap peas. So when I make a stir-fry, I set aside a handful of snap peas so that he can enjoy them raw.

9. Focus on the journey.
I would argue that as important as it is to fuel our families with nutritious foods, we have an even greater responsibility as parents to teach our kids about food choices so that they can make good decisions away from our dinner tables. Pushing one more bite of greens or two more bites of anything is not the end goal.

Don't forget that food and family meals connect us. Yes, food should be nutritious. But it should also be delicious and most definitely shared. It's not always easy to do, but when we focus more on the conversation than the number of bites of broccoli, everyone feels more relaxed.

10: Be kind to yourself and have patience.
We are all just learning, experimenting, and growing. When things don't go smoothly or are downright disastrous, be flexible and ask your troop for their ideas and help.

CHAPTER 64

TEACH YOUR CHILDREN

YOUR KIDS MIGHT give you grief about healthy food choices. I have one that almost has his PhD in it. Ha! As parents it's our responsibility to train and teach our children all that we know to give them the best chance for success in life. We would never choose for our children to suffer, but that is happening each day when we feed them foods that are anything other than starches, fruits, vegetables, legumes, nuts and seeds. They might beg for hot dogs and chocolate milk, and you might say something like, "I'm just trying to protect you from getting cancer, heart disease, diabetes, etc," and they might say, "I don't really care if I get any of those things!" The truth is they might not care because they can't possibly understand what type of pain and suffering is involved in these diseases. Keep leading by example, teaching and training them.

I'm blessed that most of my kids are totally on board with this diet; that's exciting! I know that someday all of my kids will appreciate the efforts I make to help them be the best they can be in all aspects of their lives, including their health. I know they will, and do, appreciate it.

The reason this diet is the hardest for one of my kids is because he cheats the most, so it's the hardest for him to live without junk. Rich food is addictive! I'm doing my best to teach him the WHY of how we eat. The funny part is that he really hassles me, but if anyone else eats bad food or talks about what you should or should not eat, he is the first to chime in with health stats. At least I know he is listening!

When you kids beg for junk food, try to find a healthy alternative. Do your best to work together to make healthy choices. Start by not having the junk food at home. If you are at a party or event the circumstances are a bit different. Where possible, eat first and bring healthy food to share.

Force is not the best way to go about getting your family to eat healthy, as I've learned. Lead by example, cook healthy choices, and have healthy snacks on hand. Talk and more importantly listen to your family and their ideas. Most of the time, most kids will eat what you make them, especially as time goes on and their tastes adjust to new foods.

What Forcing Kids To Eat Looks Like 20 Years Later[171]
After digging in the research I found a study published in the 2002 issue of Appetite surveying over 100 college students. Of these young adults, 70% said they had experienced forced-food consumption during childhood. Most often than not, the forcer was a parent and the common forced foods included vegetables, red meat and seafood.

The scenario goes something like this: the forcer coerces the forcee to eat the target food for reasons such as health, variety and waste. The most common tactics used were threats such as no dessert or staying at the table. In over half of these cases there was a stand-off lasting an average of 50 minutes!

What is most interesting is the internal conflict the forcees experienced — 31% experienced strong conflict, 41% moderate conflict and 29% slight conflict. Forty-nine percent said they cried, 55% experienced nausea, and 20% vomited. Most of the responses to the experience were negative with feelings of anger, fear, disgust, confusion and humiliation. The forcees also experienced feelings such as lack of control and helplessness.

Will they freely choose "that" food?
When asked if they would now eat the food they were forced to eat in childhood, 72% said they would not. The researcher's explanation is that when a child finally gives in and eats something he doesn't want to, he "loses" and the parent "wins." So later in life, when he can freely choose the food on his own, he chooses to "win."

Also, forced food consumption that results in gagging, vomiting and overall disgust can cause food aversions. Pickier kids tend to be more sensitive to different textures so being made to eat something that offends them can make that item displeasing for many years, if not a lifetime.

When asked if the forced consumption changed their overall eating habits as adults, over one-third said yes. Of those who said yes, 73% said it limited their diet and 27% said it made them more open to new foods. While this is only one study, and it does not prove cause and effect, it's important food for thought.

The Opposite Effect

After studying the feeding literature over the last few years, it's clear that many of the feeding strategies parents employ have the opposite effect. Forcing and pressuring causes kids to eat less and dislike certain foods. Restricting children makes them want to eat more.

I think a lot of it comes down to distrust. Parents have trouble believing their children will eventually learn to like a variety of foods on their own. When kids are highly food neophobic (afraid of foods), which peaks between 2 and 6, they can be very adamant about new foods, saying things like "I'll never eat that!" If a parent doesn't understand the child's development, and that this is normal and will lessen with time, they'll be more likely to fight against it making the stage last longer.

So as you can see, eating is different from other habits such as cleaning and brushing teeth. It involves taste, texture, appetite, temperament, listening and trust. It's not about making or tricking a child eat what's in front of them, but creating the circumstances that will help a child eat well today, and 20 years from now.

CHAPTER 65

COMMUNICATION

When we make changes in our diet and in our life, we need to be good at communicating with our family about the desired changes. I recently learned that I was a very poor communicator! Here are some really helpful things I've learned about communication this year from *The Five Secrets of Effective Communication* by David D. Burns, MD, from his book, *Therapist's Toolkit*.[172] His Book *Feeling Good Together*[173] really breaks down these skills so grab that book if you'd like to learn more.

LISTENING SKILLS

1. *The Disarming Technique: Seek and find some truth in what the other person is saying, even if it seems totally unreasonable or unfair to you.*
2. *Empathy: Put yourself in the other person's shoes and try to see the world through his/her eyes. a. Feeling empathy – Acknowledge how he/she is probably feeling. For example, (husband speaking), "So then the clerk told me to go to the end of the line and that was about all I could take." (wife speaking) "It sounds like that must have made you really angry." b. Thought empathy – Paraphrase the other person's words. For example, (wife speaking), "I have fourteen things to do that all have to get done by noon today, so I would love to have some help with some of this!" (husband speaking) "You have a lot of things to do today, and you could use my help right now. Is that right?"*
3. *Inquiry: Ask gentle, probing questions to learn more about what the other person is thinking and feeling. SELF-EXPRESSION SKILLS*

4. *"I Feel" Statements:* Use "I feel" statements, such as "I feel upset," rather than "you" statements, such as "You're wrong!" or "You're making me furious!"
5. *Stroking:* Find something genuinely positive to say to the other person, even in the heat of battle. Doing so conveys an attitude of respect, even though you may feel very angry with the other person at the moment.

CHAPTER 66

SHARE THE LOVE

PROBABLY ONE OF the hardest things about this diet is that I want to share it with everyone and a lot of people don't want to hear it. People suffer, complain about their health, the side effects of their medication, how awful they feel and how they can't lose weight. I have an easy answer and most people are not sure that they want to hear it. There are all sorts of reasons why people don't want to change. Most people ask the question, "if this plant based diet is really the secret, why didn't my doctor tell me this?" Doctors are not trained in nutrition. They are trying to make money and they make money with prescribing medications, office visits and surgeries. Doctors read the same studies that we hear about in magazines that are funded by agribusiness. Most doctors will tell you that meat, dairy, eggs and oils are good for you. That's the general consensus we've all been told and like most Americans, doctors believe it too. I'm excited about the doctors that get frustrated when they see that they just can't seem to heal their patients, and learn about nutrition and find the truth about how the body can heal itself when fed properly. These doctors get excited and then promote a plant based diet to their patients. These doctors are few, but the word is spreading and one day we will all know how vitally important food is for to our health. It's not our genes that cause disease. Genes load the gun but diet pulls the trigger. If you'd like to find a plant based doctor in your area, check out this web site, http://plantricianproject.org/plant-based-docs.[174]

I'm grateful for those doctors and scientists who have worked for many, many decades, promoting the whole food, plant based diet. I'm also grateful for a history of people on this planet, living on starches. I'm also grateful for a religious health code that recommends a plant based diet.

When I find a truth like this, I want to share it. It amazes me that I'd never heard about a whole food, plant based diet until I had a broken back, and found it while I was lying in bed researching health. I had heard about my religion's health code but I didn't know how to apply it, and I thought I'd just gain weight from eating all those carbohydrates/starches!

Much of the information that I've learned has been known for 100 years yet it's been kept hush hush by agribusiness industry, who are loud and in your face promoting their products. I'm happy to share what I've learned with you as it's really blessed my life, and I want to pass those blessings onto you too.

CHAPTER 67

STRIPPING GREENS

I'VE LEARNED FROM Ann Esselstyn, the wife of Dr. Caldwell Esselstyn, that you should strip some of your greens before you eat them, such as the collards and the kales. The fibrous center is pretty tough even when they're cooked. So wash them well, then grab the stem in one hand and the leaves and another and with a quick motion pull the two sides apart, removing the leaves from the stem. It's kind of fun, like tearing off a Band-Aid®, but it doesn't hurt!

Dr. Caldwell Esselstyn, the author of *Prevent and Reverse Heart Disease*[175] really promotes greens. His patients with heart disease eat greens six times per day as part of their heart disease reversal program. Greens do the opposite of fat in your veins and arteries. They expand veins, or dilate them. Eating fats contract your veins and it last for many hours. Whether you have heart problems or not, eat more greens to keep your heart healthy.

CHAPTER 68

IF IT HAS A FACE OR A MOM …

PLEASE DON'T EAT It! I watched the movie Cowspiracy[176] with my family. The movie was very eye-opening. The story is about a man who is trying to do everything he can to leave a light "footprint" on the Earth, even putting his car in storage and riding a bike, taking fast showers, etc. He then found out that what he was doing did help the Earth, but that if he would just stop eating burgers he could save 660 gallons of water per burger that he chose not to eat. He would also be saving the Earth from the methane emissions, raw sewage, and forest clearing used to grow the crops to feed the cows. Making a choice to stop eating meat had an enormous effect on the Earth, but his previous conservation efforts were really less than a drop in the bucket. This man was so excited about the new information that he found.

He wondered why he had not heard of this before. He started going to save-the-Earth-type conservation websites, and was blown away that **NOBODY** was talking about the elephant in the room. He started sending emails and making calls and visiting these groups, and again, they were focused on the mice in the room and not the elephant.

Why? He found several reasons. First, people who speak out against agribusiness wind up missing, especially in other countries. Can you believe that? I think the movie said that 1,100 people have been killed to date for speaking out about this issue. In the US, you know what happens. Look at the Texas Cattlemen vs. Oprah Winfrey six-year lawsuit.[177] It's dangerous to speak up. Isn't this the craziest thing? Watch the movie and learn why, for the Earth's sake, it's best to pet and not eat the animals. From reading my previous chapters, you know why it's best for your body to also pet and not eat the animals.

This "mama and a face" recommendation also applies to sea life. We are devastating our oceans by overfishing. Factory farms really don't help, as those farmers' fish the oceans to feed their farm fish. Also, the ocean is polluted and we eat that pollution when we eat fish. The USDA guidelines warn against methyl mercury which is found in fish. Let's stick to starches, fruits and vegetables.

CHAPTER 69

SWEET!

100% PURE ORGANIC maple syrup is a good sweetener if you have to add one to a dessert recipe or need a sweet topping for your oatmeal. Nature made delicious desserts in the form of fruit too. After some time on a plant based diet you will be amazed at how sweet and satisfying fruit for dessert is. It takes a bit of time until you're no longer accustomed to the standard American diet sweetness. I use maple syrup in all my baking instead of sugar. Make sure when you are baking that you use less liquid in your recipe to adjust for the liquid sweetener instead of the dry sugar that you are replacing.

You can also use banana as a sweetener. Make sure it's a ripe or overripe banana to get the extra sweet taste.

In my vinaigrette salad dressings I use organic unfiltered apple juice as my sweetener, or add a touch of maple syrup too. Sweet!

My next favorite sweetener is dates. My favorite strawberry pie recipe uses date as sweetener and boy, is it delicious! Check out that recipe in my recipe section.

HOMEMADE RAW DATE SYRUP[78]

This is one of the easiest recipes I have ever made! I wanted to share it with you as it is a handy natural sugar substitute this time of year. It is NOT sugar free, dates are still sugar, BUT if you are going to make something sweet, then you can at least use a natural sugar source rather than something like bleached, processed caster sugar.

Dates are a fantastic natural, raw sweetener but obviously in their normal whole form, you can't add them to everything. Turn them into a liquid however, and you have a mild tasting sugar substitute. I have used it to substitute everything from in baking to in a green smoothie or even in my cup of tea or hot chocolate.

You really need to use the Medjool dates as they are juicer and blend better. The lemon juice just helps to keep it fresh. You can also experiment with adding some vanilla extract or even some spices if you want it to be flavored. I can totally see this being gingerbread flavored in a beautiful glass jar as a gift! You can reduce the amount of water you add and you will that have a beautiful sweet date spread.

DATE SYRUP

Serves 2 cups / approx. 280 calories per 1 cup serve approx. macronutrient breakdown: fat 0g / carbs 76g / protein 2g

Ingredients
10 Medjool dates, pitted
1 3/4 cup water
1 tbsp. fresh lemon juice

Method
Place all ingredients in a blender and start the blender on a low speed to allow the dates to break up initially, and then blend on high for a few minutes until smooth. Pour into a clean glass jar and store in the refrigerator for up to 3 weeks.

Homemade Date Paste[179]
Yield: *2 Cups Date Paste*
Prep Time: *15 mins + Overnight Soak*
Ingredients:
450 Grams Pitted Medjool Dates (~1 1/3 cups)
3/4 Cup Water
1 Teaspoon Vanilla Extract (Optional)

101 THINGS I WISH I KNEW BEFORE I FED MY CHILDREN

Directions:

Place the dates in a large glass jar with a lid and add the water.

Shake well, and let sit overnight.

In the morning, place the dates and soaking water in a food processor and puree until very smooth.

Stir in the vanilla if using, and store in the refrigerator or freezer until ready to use.

CHAPTER 70

CONTRADICTION

WHY IS THERE so much contradictory information about diet and nutrition? You can read one study that says meat will give you cancer and then read another study that says how healthy animal protein is for your body. You can find these types of contradictions about many health topics.

Here's the reason: Companies are trying to sell you their products. There are accurate studies done by unbiased scientists, and there are studies done by the companies that want to sell you their food. It's quite amazing how the test results change when the company selling the product does the nutritional testing. Also, look who funded any study that you are reading. Most nutrition studies are done by the meat, dairy and egg industries as they have the most money to spend selling you their products and promoting their products. It's too bad that they are happy to tell you half-truths that sound like whole truths.

Some whole food, plant based doctors have a really hard time finding a magazine or journal to publish their studies in as most medical magazines and journals are funded by either Big Pharma or agribusinesses, and neither want the truth spoken or learned.[180] That would hurt their big company profits!

Western doctors are trained in Western medicine, which is treating the problem not finding the cause of the problem. There are basically three options: Surgery, medication or physical therapy. And if they do tell you to watch your diet they suggest the wrong diet because they're being sold the same studies the rest of us are. And really, what good is it for them to cure your heart disease with broccoli when you could give them $100,000 for heart surgery? I'm not saying that doctors are evil or greedy; they just do what they were taught to do and what pays their bills. I do believe that Western medicine goes about it all wrong; however, it's also true that we are used to this form of medicine and we want a quick fix. Maybe we would rather have heart surgery than eat broccoli; that's something to consider.

Of course there are times when we are all grateful for Western medicine, like when I broke my back and Life Flight came out to get me of the side of a mountain and shot me with morphine. I was very thankful. But I was not thankful about seven months later when doctors did a bone scan on me; I had an allergic reaction and was temporarily paralyzed for about a month. I then spent more time and money and had a lot of stress as doctors told me I had possibly developed a list of scary diseases, including MS, cancer or Guillain-Barré syndrome, not knowing my problem was that I was allergic and having a reaction to the radioactive material that they shot into my veins.

When you have cancer, diabetes, heart disease, obesity, multiple sclerosis or any disease, and even ailments like acid reflux, you can heal yourself with what you put in your mouth. The truth is out there. As always, when the student is ready, the teacher will appear.

CHAPTER 71

EAT COLORFUL

THIS CHAPTER IS dedicated to my grandma, Esther Sommer. If only I had a dollar for every time I heard her say, "Dr. Bernard Jensen says, 'eat colorful!'" as she walked around checking our plates to make sure there was enough color. Obviously, we're talking about the beautiful colors found in plant foods, not colors like you find in candy!

My grandparents were both born in Switzerland and came to America in 1949, the year my mom was born. They had a beauty school, and my grandma ended up getting really sick from all the perm solutions and different chemical products that they were using in their beauty school. My grandma decided to learn about health, and also cured her health condition by getting rid of the beauty school and learning about health. Grandma changed professions to become a masseuse. My grandparents had a huge garden and orchard. They started growing a lot of their own food, and I remember loving her white bean and vegetable soups.

When you eat a meal, your plate should be beautiful enough to take a photo of it and post it in a culinary magazine. If not, add some color and eat it. Those colors are the vitamins and minerals your body needs for optimum functioning.

Color Your World with Fruits and Vegetables[181]

Eating a rainbow of colors every day is one of Dr. Bernard Jensen's famous recommendations for keeping healthy. Every pigment provides a specific protection for plants. Research shows that humans receive similar benefits from eating colorful vegetables and fruit.

Red

Red vegetables and fruit contain a variety of phytochemicals including lycopene. Foods rich in lycopene are known for their ability to fight heart disease and some cancers, such as prostate cancer. Lycopene-rich foods include: watermelon, pink grapefruit, tomatoes and tomato-based products (spaghetti sauce, tomato paste, tomato juice, and tomato soup), papaya and guava. Use a small amount of fat, such as olive oil, when cooking tomato-based products to help the body absorb lycopene.

Find your daily dose of reds in red apples, cherries, red grapes, raspberries, watermelon, beets, strawberries, red cabbage, red onion, radishes, red peppers, rhubarb, tomatoes, chili peppers, and red potatoes.

Orange & Yellow

Orange and yellow fruits and vegetables contain powerful antioxidants such as vitamin C in addition to the phytochemicals, carotenoids and bioflavonoids. Deep orange vegetables and fruit contain beta-carotene, a disease-fighting antioxidant. Beta-carotene is believed to play a role in reducing risk of cancer and heart disease, promoting good eyesight, boosting the immune system and slowing the aging process.

Include orange and yellow fruits and vegetables in your diet every day, like yellow apples, apricots, butternut squash, carrots, corn, cantaloupe, grapefruit, lemons, mangoes, nectarines, oranges, papaya, peaches, pineapples, pumpkin, yellow peppers, and yellow raisins.

Green

Green vegetables contain potent phytochemicals such as lutein and indoles. Leafy greens are rich in energizing and alkalizing chlorophyll. Go green every day with fruits and vegetables like avocados, green apples, asparagus, artichokes, Asian greens, broccoli, Brussels sprouts, celery, cucumbers, green grapes, green beans, green cabbage, kiwi, spinach, leeks, limes, okra, pears, peas, and zucchini.

Lutein is a powerful antioxidant known for its ability to protect your eyes and maintain good vision. Green vegetables such as spinach, collards, kale,

Romaine lettuce and other leafy greens, green peas, broccoli, as well as honeydew melon and kiwi fruit, pack a lutein punch.

Indoles are believed to play a role in protecting against some cancers, such as breast and prostate. Foods rich in indoles include arugula, bok choy, broccoli, Brussels sprouts, cabbage, cauliflower, kale, rutabaga, Swiss chard, turnips, and watercres.

Blue & Purple

Blue and purple fruits and vegetables contain anthocyanins and phenolics that are powerful free radical fighters. These two antioxidants are believed to contribute towards reducing cancer and heart disease risk and slowing the aging process, in addition to having anti-inflammatory effects. The best sources of anthocyanins are beets, blackberries, black currants, blueberries, elderberries, and purple grapes. The best sources of phenolics are prunes, raisins, eggplant and fresh plums. Other sources include boysenberries, cherries, cranberries, purple asparagus, purple cabbage, purple peppers, and red grapes.

Whatever food ideas you come up with, always ask yourself, am I eating a rainbow?!

CHAPTER 72

TAKE CARE OF YOU FIRST

IF YOU'VE BEEN on an airplane, you know what the flight attendants tell you at the beginning of the flight. If the cabin loses pressure, oxygen masks will drop from the ceiling. First, place a mask over your own face and then help others around you. Why do they give that advice? You really can't lift and serve others around you if you are not oxygenated yourself. In life, there are many ways we can oxygenate ourselves in addition to breathing. Explore what fills you and do more of it!

Some people say they have too much going on. They don't have time to exercise, meditate, garden, or cook healthy foods. I say that we all have the same 24 hours in every day, and we choose what we put on our plate. Not only our dinner plate, but on our schedules. Sure, we need to make a living, but we need to keep our priorities straight so that our life is happy, healthy and enjoyable. We are in charge of our own happiness!

One time I was listening to Dr. Laura on the radio, and a lady called in saying that she was just overwhelmed with her life and all the responsibilities she had. Dr. Laura said, in her straightforward way, "So get rid of some your responsibilities." "Easier said than done" is what I was thinking, but it's so true. We have to find our own joy, and when we have so much going on that we can't even take care of ourselves, it's not beneficial to anybody. When you're healthy, it makes life a whole lot easier, more joyful and productive. Let's get happy and healthy by taking care of ourselves and then those we love around us.

7 Keys To Success On A Healthy Vegan Diet[182]

1. Make starches and fruit the basis of your diet.

Many people immediately think of broccoli or kale when they hear the words "plant-based diet." Although it's beneficial to eat leafy vegetables in abundance, they simply do not have enough calories to fuel you and satisfy your appetite (a full pound of kale, for example, has only 223 calories). To succeed on this diet, it's important that you eat enough healthy calories. This means making starches or fruit the center of your meal plate.

When making a savory meal, use foods like potatoes, sweet potatoes, whole grains, and legumes to create meals you really enjoy. Think dishes like bean enchiladas, pesto pasta, and chickpea pot pie. Contrary to urban legend, we are not talking about a diet of bok choy here—thank goodness!

2. Eat the foods you enjoy and don't worry about individual nutrients.

Many people view food as a nutritional balancing act, and they go through their day trying to make sure to get just the right amount of the countless number of nutrients out there. People are carefully calibrating their protein, carbs, lycopene, or whatever nutrient is in the news that week.

On a plant-based diet, such precision isn't necessary and the worry that comes with it can hinder your ability to stay the course. Simply choose your foods from the categories of whole fruits, vegetables, tubers, whole grains, and legumes; eat a variety across these categories over time, and eat until comfortably satiated. The most important key to success is to find or make the greatest meals you can. Nothing will help you stay on the plan more than a killer sweet-potato lasagna.

3. Don't sweat the small stuff.

Focus on the big changes like switching from meat, milk, and eggs to whole-plant foods. Such changes dramatically improve the nutritional composition of the foods you are eating, so this is where you will find the most noticeable and measurable improvements in your health.

Worrying about eating only fresh, local, or organic foods is folly when you were eating fast food and Ring Dings a few weeks ago. Since choosing whole plants is the most important thing you can do for both your health and the world around us, be sure that priority is well taken care of before seeking loftier goals.

4. Check online and call ahead when eating out.
If you're looking for a place to go, a small amount of research goes a long way—and can usually be done in just a few minutes. For example, if you're thinking about Italian food, search online to find restaurants and see what others are saying about them. Look around, read a few reviews and boom, you've found a place with multiple pasta dishes, some minestrone, and pasta e fagioli. Call and make sure the veggie options you like are vegan and can be done with no- or minimal oil—and you're on your way!

If your friends or coworkers invite you out and they already have a place in mind, check out the menu online and gauge how veg-friendly it is. If veg doesn't seem a priority, place a call ahead and let them know you are coming; the chef is almost always happy to accommodate. Let him or her know you like hearty foods like potatoes, pasta, beans and so on—this is your insurance against having your main meal be the dreaded plate of steamed asparagus.

5. Find your plant-based tribe.
Surround yourself with like-minded people who share your joy of living the plant-based life. Join groups on social media, attend local meetups, and, most importantly, make some real-life friends that share your enthusiasm.

Having people in your life that share your values will remind you of why you do what you do. It's also a great way to exchange ideas from recipes and restaurants to handling family and social situations.

6. When vacationing abroad, travel to places where it's easy to get great plant-based food.
The good news about traveling on a plant-based diet is the world is filled with places where animal-free foods are abundant. Regardless of what part of the world you are traveling to, you are likely to find some kind of plant-based fare that's ingrained in the culture and will suit your needs..

If food is as important to you as it is for me, consider what your food options will be like when making your travel plans. It's a good idea to research online to get a feel for the local vegan fare. Prior to staying in hotels or working with a guide, let your contacts know your dietary needs. You will be surprised how much they are willing to advise and help you navigate the waters.

When traveling to a place where you don't speak the native tongue, ask someone who speaks both languages fluently to help you make a "cheat sheet" of all your dietary needs. When you're out and about, just hand the small sheet of paper to your host or server—and all of your lives just became easier.

This is the "cheat sheet" I use when I travel to Thailand. It translates to: I am a vegan. I do not eat any meat. I do not eat any food that has eggs, fish sauce, oyster sauce, or milk as a part of the ingredients. I can eat garlic.

7. Be a patient advocate: Share your advice and enthusiasm when the time is right.

Our love of this lifestyle and the way it makes us feel lead us to want to shout about it from the rooftops. We want to share the message with everyone and have each person we meet adopt the lifestyle right away. And of course being a positive influence to the people around us is a noble goal!

However, as counterintuitive as it might seem, resist the urge to talk a lot about your lifestyle when meeting new people. Untimely discussions can lead to frustration and agitation, which can hurt potential friendships. Since food and health are sensitive topics, it's important to first establish commonality. For example, if you share a love of sports or hobbies, it will establish the camaraderie needed to have more open and trusting conversations later on.

When is the time right? When someone begins asking questions and does so out of genuine curiosity. With much goodwill built up from the things you have in common, you'll be on your way to making a difference in each other's lives. The more positive relationships you can associate with your plant-based way of life, the more likely you will succeed in the long run.

CHAPTER 73

EAT WHEN YOU ARE HUNGRY

THERE WERE SO many years of my life when I restricted my calories, obsessed about everything I put in my mouth, and really went hungry. For probably 12 years, I would let myself eat when I was hungry only on the weekends. And for another several years I only let myself eat vegetables after 4:00 p.m. I was tough on myself. Looking back, I feel sorry that I was so hard on myself during those times. Now I eat anytime I'm hungry and eat as much as I want, but the food I eat is satisfying, filling, delicious, low-calorie and healthy.

When you eat the food your body was made to eat, your body will function properly including keeping your weight where it should be. When you're not eating the way you should be, such as the way we're convinced to eat by the marketing of mega food companies, or because of the addictions we've formed eating chemically enhanced foods, achieving a healthy weight is a continuous struggle for most people. That is no way to live! Be willing and open to hear the truth. The truth, as they say, will set you free.

EAT WHEN HUNGRY-STOP WHEN SATISFIED[183]

Have you ever watched an infant or a child eat? It's the most fascinating thing. They eat when they are hungry and stop when they are satisfied. They do not count calories, fat grams, or amount of carbohydrates. They do not deliberately starve themselves, nor do they overeat. They listen to both their hunger and satiety cues and eat accordingly.

The older we get, the more distorted our views of eating become. We begin to control (or lose control of) our food intake, and our eating habits become anything but natural. We diet, lose weight, gain weight back, binge, starve, and then start the whole vicious cycle again. How does this craziness stop? How can people figure out when to eat and when to stop eating?

Being aware of hunger and satiety cues and eating in response to them is the first step in figuring out how much you need to eat. Hunger cues might include a feeling of emptiness, fatigue, slight irritability, or a rumbling in your stomach. Feelings of satiety can include physical satisfaction, disappearance of the hunger cues, and sudden energy. Each person experiences individual hunger and satiety cues. It's up to you to identify and become aware of when you are hungry and when you are satisfied.

A good tool to use is the hunger scale, which starts at 0 and ends at 10. The number "0" is feeling beyond hungry, lightheaded, famished, cranky, and weak. "1" is really, really hungry. "2" is really hungry. "3" and "4" are normal hunger. "5" is no feeling. "6" and "7" are satisfied. "8" is full. "9" is really full. "10" is miserably full, such as Thanksgiving dinner full.

Practice rating your hunger level before you eat and then again when you are finished eating. If you do this each time you eat, you will become more familiar with your eating patterns. When you eat in response to physical hunger, you gradually experience a sense of satisfaction. This is your body telling you that the hunger is gone. You may not be attuned to your body's signals, or you may choose to continue eating for other reasons, but then it is your mind deciding how much to eat, not your body. If you listen to your body, it will reliably "tell" you when it is hungry and when it is full.

For the most part, start eating when you are at level 3-4 and stop eating when you are at level 6-7. This is considered "normal" eating. If you find yourself consistently falling out of this range, you might want to take a good look at your eating habits. Are you eating (or not eating) for emotional reasons? Are you eating enough food to meet your physical needs? Are you in touch with your hunger and satiety cues? Do you need a more structured meal plan? Is eating a pleasant experience? All of this information is important to ensure healthy and pleasant eating.

In summary, eat when you are physically hungry and stop when you are physically satisfied. Do not allow yourself to get too hungry because that could lead to overeating later on. Do not allow yourself to overeat because that does not feel good mentally, emotionally, or physically. Put food in its place as a very small part of your life.

CHAPTER 74

SOAKING WHOLE GRAINS/BEANS/NUTS/SEEDS.

IF YOU HAVE any trouble with gluten or your digestion when you eat grains, beans, nuts or seeds, make sure you're buying organic whole grains. If you're not, start doing that first and see if that helps your digestive system. There might be some chemical on your food that is bothering your system. Another thing to try is soaking your grains before you cook them. Soaking grains, nuts, beans and seeds removes some of the phytic acid, increases nutrition and makes them more digestible.

PROS of SOAKING WHOLE GRAINS, NUTS, BEANS, and SEEDS:[184]

- *It's easy-peasy-lemon-squeezy with a little practice.*
- *It breaks down the **gluten**, phytic acid and anti-nutrients into a more digestible form.*
- *It creates the enzymes needed to digest grain properly so your body can absorb a high amount of the nutrients, minerals and vitamins that are already there.*

CONS of SOAKING WHOLE GRAINS, NUTS, BEANS, and SEEDS:

- *You have to think ahead of cooking/eating. It takes anywhere from 4-12 hours to soak whole kernels.*
- *You will feel great and develop nutrition superpowers, which will probably make your friends your family jealous.*

How Do I Soak My Whole Grains, Nuts, Beans, And Seeds?

The process is VERY simple. But the soaking times can vary depending on the grain, nut, bean or seed.

Step 1 – *Soak your grain, nut, bean or seed in water. Make sure the water is double the amount of grain, nut, bean or seed, because it will be absorbed a bit. Leave the bowl or jar on your countertop at room temperature for the specified time for your desired Soaking Food. If it calls for a long soaking time, then you'll need to change the water once or twice.*

Step 2 – *Drain the liquid and cook your grain or bean normally (it will have a shorter cooking time). Eat your nut and/or seed plain, roast them if you desire. It's safe! You can also make nut/seed milk or nut/seed butter at this point. You also have the option to dehydrate the grain, bean, nut or seed, but keep in mind that they will not last as long at room temperature and last longer frozen after they've been soaked and dehydrated.*

OPTIONAL STEP *(but a highly recommended one) – Add 1-2 TBS. Of apple cider vinegar to your water during the soaking time. This will aid in the development of phytase, the enzyme needed to break down the phytic acid found in grains, nuts, beans, and seeds.*

At my house, I mostly soak beans and not much else. Again, soaking makes them more digestible with less of your family singing the "Beans, Beans" song. Ha!

When you switch your diet, it will most likely take your body a few weeks to adjust. Don't get too worried about any digestive issues that arise temporarily. This too shall pass. No pun intended. :)

CHAPTER 75

REGROW YOUR KITCHEN VEGGIES/HERBS IN WATER

ONE OF MY favorite tips that I have been given is to regrow my green onions. Thank you, Rosette Pine for that tip! Buy five or six bunches of organic green onions from the grocery store, and as you use them, chop off about three inches from the stem and put them in a jar of water in your window sill. As long as you keep watering them, those green onions will just grow and grow and grow. The only trouble I have had is that in the hot summer the water can get a little stinky. One way around that is to plant the green onions in a little pot outside. I now have green onions growing inside, and outside, and everywhere it seems. It seems that every day I am running outside to chop some fresh green onions to go with whatever I am making. One daughter has to have them every day on her veggie sandwiches, which we pack for lunch. Yum!

Kitchen Scraps You Can Regrow With Nothing But Water[185]
Lettuce *is one of those staples that tends to get used in all kinds of meals year round so chances are you're buying a head once a week or so. Instead of tossing that heart in the trash when you're done, you can regrow new leaves.*

The next time you chop up a head of romaine lettuce for salad, hang on to the very bottom.

Take the bottom of the heart and place it in jar with about a half-inch of water. Put that in a window sill near some sunlight. Then replace the water every one or two days. Within a few days you'll have some leaves sprouting up. From there, just let the lettuce grow, trimming off any brown leaves that might wither on the outside. When you have enough green leaves sprouting up, eat away. You can do this with most other red and green lettuces as well.

Garlic sprouts are usually chopped off and thrown away as a sign you've left garlic out for too long, but they're edible if you get the right bits. They have a nice, less abrasive taste than a clove of garlic and make a good topping when they're sprouted. The initial sprout is bitter and terrible tasting, so you'll need to grow them for a bit first. If you have a garlic clove with a green sprout coming out of it, pull it aside and put in a small jar with enough water to cover the bottom of the jar. Within a couple of days, the clove will produce roots, and shortly after the sprouts will rise up to a few inches tall. When they're at least three-inches tall, you can trim off about 1/3 of the shoot.

Fennel has a strong enough taste that it's pretty rare you'll need more than just a small cutting from one. If you'd like to keep one around all the time, it's worth just regrowing one you have. Just take the bulb, put it in a cup, and fill it up with water so the bulb's covered. Stick that jar in the sun and within a few days it'll start sprouting up. Replace the water every couple of days and trim off a bit of fennel when you need it.

Leeks are awesome for soups, and it turns out they're easy to keep around because they grow in water just as easily as green onions. Just take the base of your leeks, cover them in water, and leave them in the window with some sun for a few days. You should start seeing them sprout right away, and within a week or so you'll be able to trim off parts to use in recipes.

CHAPTER 76

TO SOY OR NOT TO SOY?

I WAS NOT quite sure how simple or how complex to make this chapter. I've decided to keep it simple. If you want all the science behind my short answer, as always, Dr. John McDougall has a great article on this topic at https://www.drmcdougall.com/misc/2005nl/april/050400pusoy.htm. Or even easier, just type soy into his search feature and scroll down to see this article.

Here is what I've learned about soy. Traditional soy, like edamame, is healthy and delicious. Processed soy, the kind that you find in protein bars and processed foods is the opposite of healthy. You've probably heard bad rumors about soy; but again, we need to specify what type of soy we are talking about. It's like the difference between corn and corn oil or corn syrup. Natural corn is wonderful. Processed corn is not. Look at traditional Asians who eat more unprocessed soy than Americans. On average they live longer, are healthier and they have less reproductive issues, less cancer, less disease and hardly any hot flashes!

Processed soy is hiding in so many foods today. It's always best to buy pure and natural foods that don't come with labels. If you are buying something packaged, look for these names that mean processed soy and avoid them: defatted soy flour, organic textured soy flour, textured vegetable protein, isolated soy protein, soy protein isolates, soy protein concentrates, and soy concentrates.

The type of soy that is okay to eat, don't go crazy of course as it's high in fat and sometimes sodium, are: boiled soybeans (edamame), tofu (soybean curd), natto (fermented soybeans), miso (fermented soybean paste), okara (a by-product of tofu), soybean sprouts, soy milk, yuba (by-product of soy milk), kinako (soy flour), and soy sauce. These foods are made from simple processes like grinding, precipitation, and fermentation—thus, most of soy's ingredients remain little altered. Less than five percent of daily calories in the typical diet of Japanese or Chinese people come from soybeans.[186]"

CHAPTER 77

GOT DRUGS?

I WAS BLESSED to listen to a delightful and eye opening talk by Dr. Adriane Fugh-Berman, MD who is an Associate Professor in the Department of Pharmacology and Physiology and in the Department of Family Medicine at Georgetown University Medical Center. Dr. Fugh-Berman is shedding some light on what's really going on with prescriptions in America, and runs a non-profit group called PharmedOut[187] to educate doctors and the public about what is happening.

Dr. Fugh-Berman opened my eyes to the marketing genius of the pharmaceutical companies. She says that drug companies spend large amounts of money on their drug representatives whose job it is to schmooze doctors into prescribing more drugs. Pharmaceutical companies earn $13 for every $1 they spend on their drug representatives' salaries and expense accounts. So when Dr. Fugh-Berman says that "lunch matters" in her lecture, she is talking about the drug reps buying the doctors' lunches, among other things. Studies have found that even small gifts given to doctors, like lunch, have an effect on doctors' prescribing habits. Dr. Fugh-Berman and her team try to educate doctors about not be being bribed by the pharmaceutical companies and over-prescribing drugs to their patients.

A study was done with college students; the students were made to do a really boring task and then they were paid to tell the next group that the task was actually fun. They paid some students $200, and those students were happy to flat-out lie to the next group about the excitement of the task. Some students were only paid $5 and they still lead the next group of students to believe that the task was not that bad and kind of enjoyable.

That study helps Dr. Fugh-Berman to show that even drug reps bringing doctors a pizza makes a difference in the amount and type of drugs they prescribe. As patients, we expect our doctors to only prescribe what is necessary and best suited for us—if anything really is necessary. Many doctors are prescribing more drugs than needed and not choosing the best tied-and-true drug but instead the drug being promoted to them.

We all know that prescription drugs have side effects. There is a lot of suffering going on that is unnecessary, due to our faith in doctors and our choice to get and take any prescriptions(s) they recommend. Big pharma convinces us and our doctors that we have medical conditions that need drugs when many of these things are totally normal, like menopause, for example. Why are one in four women on hormone therapy? Because we don't feel great for whatever reason; so the doctor tells us about this new drug that might help some symptoms but it might also cause other issues, such as an increased risk of heart disease or cancer. There are drugs for too much underarm sweat, social anxiety, tiredness, binge eating, heartburn, and the list goes on and on. As human beings, we don't feel on top of the world all the time and we do have problems—and there are other ways to solve them besides medication. How about healthy diet and exercise, talk therapy, etc.? Pharmaceutical commercials actually say, "when healthy diet and exercise are not enough, try xyz drug." But what is a healthy diet? If the general public and the doctors don't know, how can they say it's not enough?

I hope we will think twice before taking medicine just because a doctor (who was most likely bribed to prescribe), wrote you a prescription. Remember that in the US, the fourth leading cause of death is accidents and the majority of those accidents are accidental poisoning. How do you become poisoned? Taking a pharmaceutical that kills you is one way.

One very surprising thing for me was the directions on my pain killers after my back surgery. The directions said that if I had adverse reactions to the medication I should KEEP TAKING THE PRESCRIPTION AND TALK TO MY DOCTOR. Wait, what? How can you not say that profit does not have something to do with those instructions? That being said, I do know there are benefits, even life-saving benefits that are found in prescription medication. However, we all know about the terrible side effects and so many of them can be avoided. Plus, when have you ever felt truly vibrant on medication? I never have.

Your health starts with you. Don't wait for a doctor to explain it to you. It's your job to learn, listen and understand yourself. You are your own best advocate. No one understands you like you do. Now that you have learned so much about health, realize that you have the power to prevent and even reverse disease by what you choose for your next bite. Choose wisely.

CHAPTER 78

THE GLYCEMIC INDEX

I CAN'T EAT carbs; they spike my blood sugar and make me fat—right?

I think the glycemic index (GI index) is totally misunderstood and misused. Let's start our discussion with what the GI index website[188] states: *The glycemic index (GI) is a ranking of carbohydrates on a scale from 0 to 100 according to the extent to which they raise blood sugar levels after eating. Foods with a high GI are those which are rapidly digested and absorbed and result in marked fluctuations in blood sugar levels. Low-GI foods, by virtue of their slow digestion and absorption, produce gradual rises in blood sugar and insulin levels, and have proven benefits for health. Low GI diets have been shown to improve both glucose and lipid levels in people with diabetes (type 1 and type 2). They have benefits for weight control because they help control appetite and delay hunger. Low GI diets also reduce insulin levels and insulin resistance.*

Recent studies from the Harvard School of Public Health indicate that the risks of diseases such as type 2 diabetes and coronary heart disease are strongly related to the glycemic index of the overall diet. In 1999, the World Health Organization (WHO) and Food and Agriculture Organization (FAO) recommended that people in industrialized countries base their diets on low GI foods in order to prevent the most common diseases of affluence, such as coronary heart disease, diabetes and obesity.[189]

Before telling you why I don't agree with the statements on this website, I should first say that I believe in the measurement method, just not in the conclusion that we should eat low GI foods for maximum health. Our bodies are made to live on starches, which are high GI foods. We know what humans have eaten for tens of thousands of years. People have been lean and strong and didn't have cancer, heart disease, diabetes, high blood pressure, high cholesterol etc. We know what happens when people switch to a high GI diet, diseases are prevented or reversed. Now by high GI, I mean whole plant based foods, not jelly donuts. Next, we know that humans have an abundance of enzymes that breaks down sugars and uses them for energy. Why would we have an abundance of the enzyme, amylase, if we didn't need to break down large amounts of glucose found in starches? Raising our blood sugar by eating triggers us to feel full and satisfied, turning off our desire to overeat and go searching for sweets. We also know that low GI foods like meat turn on cancer and heart disease.

While eating low GI foods does cause weight loss, it's not because it's good for you. Eating an abundance of animal products makes your body stop functioning properly, making you sick and causing weight loss. I can just hear someone reading this who wants to lose weight saying, "I don't care about my health, I just want to lose weight. Sign me up for the low GI diet." Please don't say that. Here is the reason: You can eat a delicious, filling, nutritious and healthy diet of starches, fruits and veggies and you will lose 8-12 pounds per month and regain your health on a high GI diet. Please don't give up your health for your waistline.

It's interesting to me that on the GI website it says that a low GI diet helps with controlling sugar levels for diabetics. That's nice, but did you know that you can cure type 2 diabetes in 10 days on a plant based diet? I don't know about you, but if I had diabetes, I'd rather cure if for the rest of my life instead of trying to control it with low GI foods.

Please forget about the GI index. It was not created for your health. It was created to measure the glucose in foods, which it does accurately. Let's not take this measurement and connect it with our health.

CHAPTER 79

SPICE IT UP

I LOVE JALAPENOS! I love basil! I love parsley! I love green onions! I love chilies! I love garlic! Don't make boring food while avoiding health problems. Grow some spices, peppers, herbs and onions in your garden and add them to all your dishes. Life is too short to eat boring food! Spice it up.

Not only are spices yummy, they are good for you. My mom's parents are from Switzerland. They used to make my mom wear a garlic clove around her neck to keep germs away from her. My mom would say it kept the people away too, which is why she never got sick. Poor mom.

Nature is perfect and has all we need for optimal health. Learn the benefits of herbs and spices and use them in your cooking.

Here are 20 great herbs and spices for your cooking and health pleasure:[190]

1. Turmeric—has anti-inflammatory and anti-cancer properties.
2. Rosemary—boosts your immune system, improves circulation, helps stomach aches and digestion.
3. Basil—strengthens cells, calms inflammation; it's good for your heart and antibacterial.
4. Cumin—aids in digestion, helps prevent diabetes and diabetic symptoms, and provides essential minerals like phosphorus, thiamine and potassium.
5. Nutmeg—cleans the liver and kidneys with its detoxifying properties, aids sleep, and helps digestion.

6. Saffron—use the extract, not the seasoning to help with depression, menstrual cramping and even degenerative diseases like Alzheimer's.
7. Ginseng—bolsters the immune system, helps mental focus and concentration, and helps general well-being.
8. Cardamom—improves indigestion, upset stomach and heartburn, fights free radical damage from toxins, lowers blood pressure because it's rich in fiber, and it's a diuretic.
9. Curry—has anti—inflammatory, anti-cancer properties.
10. Thyme—a great antioxidant; cancer and heart disease prevention, protects your cells from free radicals, and it's an antimicrobial which keeps your body free from bacteria and fungi.
11. Cayenne pepper—has detoxifying effects, calms digestion, has a cleansing effect and eradicates fungi.
12. Licorice root—calms your mood.
13. Oregano—contains minerals, fiber and omega 3.
14. Cilantro—cleans the body of toxicity from heavy metals; also, cilantro is calming and improves the ability to fall asleep and stay asleep.
15. Lavender—contains phytonutrients and enhances foods' flavor.
16. Sage—anti-inflammatory, and antioxidant rich.
17. Ginger—has been found in studies to stop and kill cancer cells.
18. Cinnamon—antiseptic, cleans the body of bacteria, improves cholesterol, is an anti-inflammatory, helps with weight loss, regulates blood sugars, and boosts metabolism.
19. Parsley—immune booster, soothes pain, full of vitamin C, good for heart health, and contains vitamin B.
20. Fennel—contains antioxidants, vitamin C, boosts the immune system, and is good for heart and eye health.

CHAPTER 80

EATING ANIMALS IS AS BAD FOR YOU AS...

...SMOKING, SAYS DR. Greger[191]. I listened to a fabulous lecture by Dr. Michael Greger via my computer from the McDougall Advanced Study Weekend, February 2016. Dr. Greger listed the top 15 causes that Americans die from and showed studies that proved that a plant based diet could prevent, reverse and even cure most of these 15 causes: heart disease, cancer, emphysema, stroke, accidents, Alzheimer's, diabetes, nephritis (kidney failure), flu, depression, blood infections, liver disease, high blood pressure, Parkinson's and pneumonia. Dr. Greger is a master of reading health studies, pulling out the truth, and sharing it with us on his free website www.nutritionfacts.org.[192] Besides the convincing studies he shares, I was inspired by the story of his grandma. At age 65 his grandma, Frances Greger, had terrible heart disease and could no longer walk due to crushing chest and leg pain. She found her way to Dr. Pritikin, and immediately adopted his whole food, plant based low fat plan, and within three weeks she was walking 10 miles per day! Frances lived another 31 years to the age of 96. Her grandson, Dr. Michael Greger, was fascinated with how her healthy diet changed her life so quickly and drastically and that was his inspiration to go into medicine.

Dr. Greger speaks about how popular smoking was in the 1950's in America. Everyone was smoking and people didn't realize how bad it was for you. They even thought it was good for you to smoke. Even doctors recommend smoking to their patients to cure all sorts of aliments. But then people started getting sick and studies were done; and guess what, after only 25 years and 7000 studies the Surgeon General had to tell America that smoking was no longer recommended. Interestingly enough, the American Medical Association did not agree with the Surgeon General. This could have had something to do with the fact that the Association received a ten million dollar gift from the tobacco industry![193] And 10 million was even more back then.

People were hearing that smoking was not safe and started to quit. How many people was it too late for, the ones that had already developed cancers and emphysema? Dr. Greger compared the smoking of the 1950's to the animal product eating of today. Who in our society eats animal products today? Almost everyone! Who recommends that we eat animal products? Government, schools, public programs, doctors, TV, radio, magazines, everyone! Probably even your mother! But guess what? This is just like the cigarettes. Please stop smoking now! Or in other words, please stop eating animal products. They are killing you, your family, your children and the planet as we've discussed in other chapters. You can turn away from the truth or embrace it. It's up to you.

How about moderation? How about cutting down on animal product intake? Is that good? Sure. It's especially good for that one animal you just didn't eat! But is it good enough for your health or the Earth? No! It's back to our same smoking analogy. Is it good enough to smoke less? Yeah, that's nice, but it's nothing like quitting all the way to preserve your health.

With 6,000-7,000 health studies coming out each year, I'm grateful to Dr. Greger for helping us to understand what these studies mean, and who funded and wrote them. I highly recommend you check out some of the studies on Dr. Greger's website, www.nutritionfacts.org.[194]

CHAPTER 81

ARE HUMANS DESIGNED TO EAT MEAT?

Dr. Milton Mills gave a superb and convincing lecture at the McDougall Advanced Study Weekend in February 2016[195], which I watched online. Dr. Milton Mills explaining that we are herbivores from head to toe. He compared our body structure to carnivores. I hope my notes can do his talk justice.

Dr. Mills started by discussing the shapes of the bodies of carnivores. Carnivores have a streamlined body shape with their organs protected on their underside as they walk on four legs. Their teeth come first when approaching them, as teeth are their first line of defense; and they can run at 35 miles per hour. Their skeleton is made so that they are always on their toes, like the ready, set, go position. They have sharp nails and claws and permanently flexed joints for rapid acceleration. They have light limbs and small feet to conserve energy. They have super-acute hearing and ears that swivel like radars. Their eyes are optimized for night vision, and to track movement and detect weak or injured prey. Their sense of smell is 100,000 times greater than ours. They can smell prey at great distances and can smell cancers, infections and disorders in easy targets. Carnivores have multiple litters and short gestation periods. Carnivore infants are born with their eyes closed and complete their fetal maturation outside the womb. Carnivore milk is 2-10 times more fattening than human milk and contains a lot more protein. Human milk has more sugar as human infants' brains are larger and need sugar to develop instead of fat and protein. Carnivores can reduce their facial muscles to allow for big bites. Their jaw muscles are very large. Carnivores don't chew their food, as their saliva has no enzymes to break down their food. Their jaws have minimal side to side motion and cannot move forward. The jaw joint is on the same plane as the teeth so they can cut through tough hides. Human bite force is 135-150 pounds per square inch (psi) while carnivores' jaw strength is 300-1000 psi.

Carnivore jaw joints are above the cheek teeth and act like a nutcracker. Our jaw moves from side to side for easy grinding and chewing. Our tongue is thick and muscular to aid in chewing. The shapes of our teeth are flatter for grinding and shredding fibrous plants and less jagged. Carnivore molars slide past each other vertically while ours slide across each other horizontally. Our small mouth creates a vacuum so we can suck while carnivores lap to drink. A carnivore's esophagus is wide and an herbivores is narrow. Ninety percent of people who choke to death choke on meat. Proteins and fat digest quickly and easily so carnivores have short digestive tracts, unlike the long elaborate tract of herbivores. Carnivore stomachs are acidic, even able to dissolve bones. Their stomachs are extremely large. They can eat up to 30% of their body weight in one meal. They are designed for intermittent feeding. Carnivores can eat putrefying, bacteria/toxin-laden flesh. Carnivores cannot absorb or digest high carb meals.

Plant protein, fat and carbohydrates have a fibrous cell wall which requires a more elaborate GI tract for digestion, like humans have. Herbivores have an unlimited capacity for carbohydrate digestion and absorption. Carnivore colons are short and straight and its only function is elimination not absorption because meat will putrefy and release toxic metabolites if not quickly eliminated. An herbivore colon is long and pouched and also helps with fermentation of fiber, water absorption, vitamin production by bacteria and enhances immune function.

Human saliva contains the enzyme amylase which breaks down carbohydrates. Gastro-esophageal reflux disease (GERD) is due to or exacerbated by diets high in fat and meat. Untreated GERD can cause cancer of the esophagus. Human stomachs are moderately acidic, hold less than one liter and we can only eat 800-1270 calories in one meal, less than our daily caloric needs. Did I mention that a wolf can eat up to 21,000 calories in one meal?

During the Stone Age there were no large scale preservation methods so hunting was not an efficient way of obtaining energy. Throughout human history, crop failures have led to famine, death and the starvation of whole populations.

The human small intestine is extremely long, 25-35 feet, characteristic of an herbivore. The small intestine is also covered with villi which look like fingers, increasing the surface area of the intestine. If you laid out the surface area of your intestine, it's about the size of a singles tennis court.

The human colon is extremely long and pouched and we have an appendix. The primary functions of the colon are: water absorption, fermenting fiber, producing short chain fatty acids, vitamin production and elimination. Food spends more time in the human colon than the stomach and small intestines combined. Fermentation of fiber in the colon generates short chain fatty acids that are vital to normal human physiology. Low fiber diets predispose us to a number of health problems and diseases. Remember, there is zero fiber in animal products.

Activation of phytoestrogens (plant derived estrogen) and lignans (chemical compounds found in plants) bring these benefits:

- Breast cancer reduction by 22% in women with the highest lignan intake.
- Whole rye grains reduce prostate specific antigen (PSA) in men with prostate cancer by 14%.
- Soy phytoestrogen reduces breast cancer risk in a dose-dependent fashion. That's like "an apple a day keeps the doctor away," but instead, some whole soy, like edamame, a day keeps cancer away. Do not eat processed soy. That does the opposite!
- Metabolism of phytoestrogens in the colon can make them more bioavailable.

There are microbes in your gut which help with immune function and reduce inflammation. When your microbes can't do their job because most eat people a diet they were not designed to eat, we get increased inflammation, less effective fermentation of fiber, and lower production of neurotransmitters like GABA, serotonin and others. Leaky gut also comes from a poor diet and relates to depression. Those with leaky gut are about two or more times more likely to have issues with major depression. Studies have shown that one meal high in animal fat can induce endotoxemia. Bacterial endotoxins increase total body inflammation and enter the body through the leaky gut. These bacteria come from meat whether it's cooked or not.

In the 2012 Alzheimer's Association Disease Facts and Figures sheet, it shows a steady increase in Alzheimer's with per capita increase in meat and animal food consumption when compared worldwide, country by country. You can guess where the U.S. is for meat and animal product consumption and also for the number of Alzheimer's cases.

In dementia patients, the higher their body inflammation, the higher the degree of dementia. Some scientists believe that they can predict cognitive decline due to the inflammatory markers. Again, the fermentation of fiber in the colon is essential for normal physiology, optimal health and brain function and protection.

Do carnivores worry about the side effects of eating fat and cholesterol? No! Here is why:

- Carnivores do NOT develop heart disease, no matter how much they eat.
- Carnivores do not develop gallstones due to excess cholesterol etc. because of the emulsifying properties in their gallbladder.
- Carnivores can detoxify vitamin A and manufacture vitamin C. They don't need to eat plants for these purposes.
- Carnivores produce urine 2.5 times more concentrated than humans. Their bodies can handle all the acidity.

- Carnivores can metabolize excess animal protein without damaging their bones.

Herbivore Physiology:

- Only herbivores have carbohydrate digesting enzymes in their saliva.
- Only herbivores have an appendix.
- An appendix is part of the GI immune system.
- Cannot detoxify vitamin A.
- Can detoxify a wide range of plant alkaloids.
- Can make vitamin A from beta-carotene
- May require a dietary source of vitamin C.
- Cannot eat rotting flesh.
- Easily develop heart disease when fed diets high in saturated fat and cholesterol.
- Can ferment fiber into beneficial short chain fatty acids.

Got Osteoporosis?
Many plant foods are abundant in calcium. Cows get enough calcium from green plants and moose and deer grow antlers of solid bone (80lbs) weighing more than an entire human skeleton (35lbs) in only three months from a diet of only plant foods.

We need to take our own health and the health of our family into our own hands. Our country is not diseased and dying for no good reason. We've been fooled into believing that we need animal products and it's killing us and there is a very easy answer to fix the health of our country. We just need to be opened minded, curious and willing to change.

I loved Dr. Milton Mills' entire lecture! It was so eye opening to understand the differences in herbivore vs. carnivore anatomy.[196] Dr. Mills used an analogy from the Bible to again help us understand that the answer is so simple that we think it can't possibly be true but it is.

When Naaman,[197] commander of the Syrian army, but also a leper, was told to wash in the river seven times, he tried to dismiss the advice because he thought it could not be that simple to be healed and he wanted the King to cure him. He did not want to take advice from a prophet. Luckily his servant convinced him to follow the Prophet Elisha's words and washed in the river seven times which healed Naaman. Health is that simple too. All the secrets to health are right before our very eyes. We go to great lengths and suffer great pains and spend fortunes on our health when there is a much simpler way that really works better than any of man's ways. Go wash in the river my friends, by eating a plant based diet.

CHAPTER 82

THE CURE FOR ACNE

Do you have acne? Do your teenagers have acne? Do you know you that can cure it with a plant based diet? You have to cut out oils too! Follow this diet for 30 days and no more pimples. Cheat and the pimples start coming back in one day. I've tried this method with myself and my teens and it works!

Do you know that there has only been one study[198] done, in 1969, to see if food has an effect on acne? The results showed that food did not have an effect on acne—but they tried the wrong food. The study took 30 people with acne and gave half of them chocolate bars with no chocolate in them—but still filled with fat—and the other participants ate regular chocolate bars. Guess what, no changes in the acne when you take out the chocolate. Since no studies have been done since then, your dermatologist will probably tell you that food does not play a part in your acne. Wrong! Stop eating fats and oils and the pimples will leave you.[199]

Here is what you have to avoid to get rid of acne:

Animal products
Nuts, seeds, avocados
Oils
Packaged foods
Vegan processed foods
Soy fake meats and cheeses

CHAPTER 83

KNOW YOUR NUMBERS

WHEN I TELL people that I don't eat animal products or oils they look at me with concern, because how can I be alive, standing and breathing yet just eating plants? I think they are thinking of broccoli, and I'm thinking of a big plate of mashed potatoes, gravy and veggies. I was curious about my numbers so I went and had my blood tested. I was especially curious about what my cholesterol was since I'm eating no animal products, and also wondered what my B12 level was, as it's a bacteria from animals that I'm not eating. I did buy some B12 supplements, but I had not taken them as I felt great and thought there was no need to take them yet as I was new to plant based eating. All my numbers came back great. My cholesterol was 62/38. The nurse had a fun time trying to make sense of that one! My B12 was in the normal range too. Very interesting! Blood pressure and all was great. I feel great too. No issues like I used to get. No more stomach aches or intestinal upset, no more body odor, bad breath, stinky feet, hardly any pimples, no more fighting my weight, no more worry of disease. What a wonderful way to live! I've also gained a wonderful new passion, to share this info with you!

The downside to knowing my numbers was the cost. It didn't even occur on me that my insurance would not cover these tests when I wanted to have them, as the doctor didn't need to order them for any reason other than my request. Get a price before you get any blood tests. It was several hundred dollars that I was not expecting to be charged.

***Track Your Progress*[200]**
Whenever possible, track at least the following basics: your weight, your blood pressure and blood test results, including the five measures below, plus any additional recommendations from your doctor.

- **Cholesterol***: If your level is above 180 mg/dl, you should consider it a warning sign of potential circulatory problems. Ideal is below 150 mg/dl. Sometimes results are broken down into HDL ["good"] and LDL ["bad"] cholesterol levels, but I feel total cholesterol is the most significant.*
- **Triglycerides***: This measures the amount of fats floating in your blood. Your level will likely be between 50 and 200 mg/dl. Higher levels indicate "sludge" in your blood, cause resistance to insulin activity, and are associated with an increased risk of heart disease.*
- **Glucose (blood sugar) level***: Normal fasting level is between 70 and 100 mg/dl. Higher levels indicate prediabetes or diabetes.*
- **BUN (Blood Urea Nitrogen)***: This level reflects the amount of protein you eat and the function of your kidneys. Normal is less than 15 mg/dl.*
- **Uric acid level***: Normal is less than 7 mg/dl. A higher figure indicates a risk of developing gout and/or kidney stones.*

CHAPTER 84

BOSOM FRIEND

"Diana Barry, will you be my bosom friend?" I love Anne Shirley from Anne of Green Gables, and I was always jealous of her and her best friend Diana Barry because I wanted a bosom friend too. It took me 35 years to find my Diana; but I finally did, and it was so worth the wait!

Sometimes, as grown-ups, we don't take enough time to be with our friends. In that, we are doing ourselves a huge disservice. Friends fill our souls with joy, laughter, love and comfort. I was at a funeral recently, and I heard a quote that "the only way to take sorrow out of death is to take love out of life." I thought that was so beautiful, and so true. Do we avoid loving because we are afraid of loss? Open your heart and let your love flow towards others. Friendship is such a blessing.

Friends are great for helping to keep you on track with your goals, and are also great exercise partners! Have some fun and burn a few calories along the way. You can garden, cook and create healthy recipes with your friends too. Your heart will be better for it in more ways than one.

Thank you to my bestie Kelli Russell for always being there for me! Just the thought of her gives me a warm, fuzzy feeling in my heart. She listens and cares and spends time with me like no one else. I am so blessed to have her in my life. She also happens to be the best yoga instructor on the planet, which I love! She's the bomb.com as my kids say! Next time you are in San Diego, take a class from Kelli. Look around for me because I will probably be there. I love yoga and there really is no better teacher in all the world then Kelli! Find Kelli's teaching schedule at www.KelliRussell.com[201] or www.yogaboost.co,[202] where she brings yoga to your office. She also mentors yoga teachers. Awesome!

CHAPTER 85

UNAWARE

My eyes were opened to what's really going on with our planet when I heard a lecture from Dr. Richard Oppenlander.[203] He wrote a book called *Comfortably Unaware*.[204] He spoke of how we are literally destroying the Earth because of our demand for animal products. We are replacing forests with pastures, adding uncountable amounts of greenhouse gas emissions into the air from animal farms, far more than all transportation combined, depleting our oceans and killing off thousands, even tens of thousands of species per year as the Earth warms from our demand to eat animals. Of course we are killing ourselves too but for this chapter let's take the focus off of us and look at the bigger picture.

Although countries are meeting and speaking and trying to figure out what they can do to stop this process of Earth destruction, they are focused on the wrong solutions. Their ideas are too expensive, too slow and they are completely ignoring the main problem. They focus on fuel emissions instead of the real issue, raising and slaughtering 70 billion animals per year and the effects of that process. How about we talk about the elephant in the room? We could all stop eating meat and the destruction of the Earth would stop immediately. But we could not ask people to do that right? I mean, where will they get their protein? That protein part is a joke, by the way, because you get all the protein you need from plant food; but the animal protein myth is believed and followed, and the meat industry is happy about that. It's sad; but really, the population as a whole does not care what they are doing to the Earth or their bodies. People want what they want, and don't care the cost to themselves or the planet. There are some people that might make changes if they were aware of the truth. I was one of them. I ate the SAD (Standard American Diet) just like most people until I learned better.

So what about the buzz words, sustainability, grass fed, natural, organic, farm-to-table etc. All these ideas don't help our planet. Grass fed actually takes more land and resources and raises the greenhouse gasses. The emissions from transporting food are small compared to the emission from growing animals to slaughter.

Let's talk about water. If you live in California like me it's a scarce commodity! According to Dr. Oppenlander in 2016, it takes 1,800 to 4,200 gallons of water to produce one pound of beef, 1,500 gallon of water to produce a pound of pork, 800 gallons of water per pound of chicken, 1000 gallons per gallon of milk, 60 gallons per egg. I was so shocked when I heard these numbers. Wow. Compare that to the water savings from producing fruits, vegetables and grains. 6 gallons per pound of carrots, 10 gallons per pound of blueberries, 34 gallons per pound of potatoes, 31 gallons per pound of most greens, 28 gallons per pound of tomatoes, 100-130 gallons for a pound of most grains. Can you imagine how much water we'd save if we ALL stopped eating animal products today?

It's amazing to know that we raise 70 billion animals for slaughter each year. Some animals need up to 60 times as much water as people do per day. And that's just for drinking. Imagine how much more water is used when we also consider the water used for growing their food, cleaning up after them and slaughtering them. More than half of all the water used in the United States goes to livestock which makes those numbers on extreme water usage in the previous paragraph make sense.

How about our oceans? According to the Food and Agriculture Organization of the United Nations, they say that approximately 70 percent of fish are either exploited or depleted. There are 1081 fish species that are endangered and we are catching fish at a rate that is three times more than what is sustainable. Dr. Oppenlander reminds us that these numbers do not consider bykill, which are the animals caught and discarded while fishing for the ones the fishermen want. For every pound of shrimp there are over 20 pounds of other sea creatures killed in the process like dolphins, turtles etc. So why don't the fishermen stop? Because we want to eat fish! We need our Omega 3s, right? Guess where fish get their Omega 3s? From plants, and so can we.

Out of sight, out of mind is what I think of when it comes to our rainforests. Seventy percent of the Amazon rainforests have been lost to cattle ranching. Ninety-five percent of Brazil's Atlantic Coast rainforest has been lost mostly to raise cattle. Every year, 34 million more acres of rainforest are lost and this has been happening since about 1970. Twenty percent of the Earth's oxygen is produced in the rainforests while taking out tons of carbon dioxide. We are destroying plant and animal species, as well as people of the Amazon, by destroying our rainforests.

Methane concentration has increased 150% since 1800. Our greenhouse gases are higher than they have been in 650,000 years of Earth's history. There are 60 billion more animals than people on earth that all breathe in oxygen and breathe out carbon dioxide. Animals also produce 89,000 pounds of pee and poop per second! YUCK! Not to mention the methane, ammonia, and nitrous oxide overload happening too. Livestock constitutes 80% of all fossil fuel emissions. Please realize what you are doing to our air when you eat meat.

This is really just the tip of the iceberg of what we are doing to our Earth because of our demands to eat animal products. I very highly recommend you read *Comfortably Unaware* by Dr. Richard Oppenlander.[205] What an eye opener.

YOU have a choice. You can eat animals that are mostly treated inhumanely while ruining your own health and our Earth, or you can choose plant based food that will give you vibrant health, has no adverse effects on you, the Earth or other living creatures. It's your choice. Vote with your next bite.

CHAPTER 86

YOUR BODY ABSORBED IT!

ARE YOU USING products filled with chemicals on your body, face, hands, hair, and teeth, such as deodorant, hand soap, laundry soap, sunscreen, lipstick, and chap sticks? What about chemicals on your furniture, counters, tables and bathrooms? Stop poisoning your family! When you put something on your skin and then it's gone, where did it go? Your body absorbed it. Be careful!

Shampoo Ingredients To Avoid
When shopping for shampoo or conditioner, always check the product labels. Just because chemicals are toxic doesn't mean they aren't used. For example, did you know that sodium lauryl sulfate is known to cause cataracts in adults and improper eye development in children? Regardless, it's a common ingredient in most varieties of shampoo and conditioner. In addition to being common, the following ingredients are known to dry out the scalp, irritate oil glands, corrode hair follicles, and are best avoided.

Sodium lauryl sulfate
Ammonium lauryl sulfate
Derivatives of lauryl alcohol
Myreth sulfate
Propylene glycol (also known as antifreeze)
Olefin sulfonate (deodorized kerosene)

The Benefits Of Organic Shampoo and Conditioner:
Ingredient quality is the primary difference between organic and conventional hair care products. Think of it as natural vs. synthetic. Organic products gently

infuse your hair follicles and skin cells with natural minerals, herbal extracts, and oils. Natural ingredients such as organic tea tree can help address skin conditions such as dandruff and scalp irritation. Beta glucan is another ingredient that helps sooth an irritated scalp.

If you are looking for shampoo that stimulates healthy hair, look for products that contain aloe vera and coconut oil as they are natural moisturizers. If you need enhanced shine, choose something with organic shea butter.

When you use organic shampoos and conditioners, you're also helping the environment by letting biodegradable substances go down the drain instead of harsh chemicals.[206]

The Benefits Of Organic Laundry Detergent

Organic laundry detergent is the best for your health. Many commercial varieties of laundry detergent contain pollutants, chemicals, and artificial preservatives, all toxic to human health.

The dirty truth behind clean clothes

If you look at the ingredient label on most commercial laundry detergents, you'll probably notice that surfactants are listed. This ingredient is a wetting agent that helps water to penetrate fabrics. The term "surfactants" isn't simply one ingredient but a reference to a number of different chemical ingredients. Surfactants can release benzene, a toxin linked to cancer and reproductive disorders.

The puzzling thing is that many of the chemicals that are used in brand name detergents aren't really geared toward keeping our clothes clean. In fact, most detergents are simply aesthetic enhancers, only improving the smell and appearance of clothing. Don't think the rinse cycle will protect you either — the ingredients in these detergents are known to agitate our health and can contribute to allergies.

What you can do

The answer is simple: use organic laundry detergent.

Organic laundry detergent does not contain chlorine, phosphates, and other artificial additives that are dangerous to human health. They are also free of synthetic dyes and perfumes, both of which can cause allergic reactions in some people and skin outbreaks in others.

Chemicals found in conventional laundry detergent emit fumes that are constantly inhaled throughout the day. Breathing in chemical fumes, even at minute concentrations, may have damaging consequences on endocrinological and neurological health. When you use organic laundry soap, you and your family are avoiding those dangers.

Phosphate, a common chemical added to laundry detergent, has significantly damaged the environment over the past 40 years. The use of phosphates in detergents has been increasingly scrutinized, mostly due to their poisonous effects on fish and the environment. Choosing organic detergent can help reduce the chemicals that invade our natural landscape.

In direct response to consumer demand, many manufacturers are attempting to go green with their products in an effort to protect the environment and satisfy their customers. Also, many laundry detergents are now being sold in smaller, concentrated forms, which some may say can reduce waste. However, the best alternative for environmental and physical health is to purchase organic detergents that are made with natural, certified ingredients. They are more gentle on fabrics, healthier for our bodies, and safer for every living thing.[207]

WHY YOU SHOULD A USE NATURAL DEODORANT

Not all deodorants are good for you. Learn which ingredients to look out for and where you can find safe and effective deodorants.

Embracing natural beauty goes beyond creams, moisturizers, lotions and makeup—it encompasses anything we put in and on our bodies, including deodorants and antiperspirants. Although we may be proud to toss out body-care products made with harsh ingredients, few of us are willing to compromise on the topic of body odor. Lack of knowledge and a fear of stinky armpits—a subject no one wants to talk about—may make you shy away from natural deodorants. But you shouldn't disregard the concerns surrounding some of the ingredients in conventional deodorants and antiperspirants. Every day we slather these products under our arms, an area where many lymph nodes lie close to the surface of the skin. And even though these products effectively block sweat and odor, many of the popular drugstore brands are loaded with questionable ingredients that are worth examining, if not also replacing, with safe alternatives.

Analyzing Aluminum

Aluminum is the active ingredient antiperspirants rely on to keep our underarms fresh. This is how it works: Aluminum salts—in the form of aluminum chloride, aluminum zirconium, aluminum chlorohydrate and aluminum hydroxybromide—prevent us from sweating when aluminum ions are drawn into the cells that line the sweat ducts, causing the cells to swell and squeezing the ducts closed so sweat cannot get out. Unfortunately, aluminum is also a known neurotoxin that has been linked to breast cancer and neurological disorders such as Alzheimer's disease. Let's briefly break down these risks. Most breast cancers develop in the upper outer part of the breast—the area closest to the armpit—and some research has suggested that aluminum compounds absorbed by the skin may cause changes in the estrogen receptors of breast cells. In addition, high levels of aluminum have been found in the brains of people with Alzheimer's disease, and a recent study from Saint Louis University found that aluminum may cause liver toxicity, a contributing factor to degenerative diseases such as Alzheimer's disease.

Aluminum-Free Deodorants

The most troubling risk factor for many of these ingredients—especially aluminum—is long-term exposure. Although studies about such health risks are not yet definitive, it makes sense to investigate safe alternatives. Fortunately, as more information comes to light about these chemical ingredients, more companies are developing safer alternatives, and with more products come more options. It's becoming easier than ever to turn to safe, effective alternatives. Here are a few types of safe products that you will find on the market.

Crystal deodorant stones contain a naturally occurring form of aluminum made up of molecules too large to be absorbed by the skin. This helps to make these products effective at preventing the odor found in sweat from developing, rather than artificially clogging pores as antiperspirants do.[208]"

HAZARDOUS HOUSEHOLD CLEANERS

Though many assume that some government agency oversees the safety of the multi-billion-dollar household cleaning products industry, it is largely unregulated. All those common chemical cleaners that require gloves to use and that we lock up from the kids? They undergo minimal scrutiny; what's a consumer to do?

Environmental Working Group (EWG) to the rescue. The watchdog organization has cast plenty of research on the toxins in everything from cosmetics to food, and are now taking household cleaners to task. 2012 was the first comprehensive independent scientific analysis of toxic chemicals in more than 2,000 cleaning products and 200 brands.

"Cleaning your home can come at a high price – cancer-causing chemicals in the air, an asthma attack from fumes or serious skin burns from an accidental spill," said Jane Houlihan, EWG senior vice president for research and co-author of the EWG Cleaners Hall of Shame. "Almost any ingredient is legal and almost none of them are labeled, leaving families at risk. Our Hall of Shame products don't belong in the home."

All in all, it's a nasty group of products, a real bunch of thugs, that really should be avoided. Here are the worst of the worst, worthy of a shout-out from the Cleaners Hall of Shame:

1. Mop & Glo Multi-Surface Floor Cleaner
A dose of methoxydiglycol (DEGME) with your shiny floor? DEGME is "suspected of damaging the unborn child" by the United Nations Economic Commission for Europe. DEGME levels in this product are up to 15 times higher than allowed in the European Union.

2. Comet Disinfectant Cleanser Powder EWG found that this scouring powder emitted 146 different chemicals, including some thought to cause cancer, asthma and reproductive disorders. The most toxic chemicals detected – formaldehyde, benzene, chloroform and toluene – are not listed on the label. Little is known about the health risks of most of the contaminants found.

3. Simple Green Concentrated All-Purpose Cleaner
Marketing claims this to be "non-toxic," but it contains 2-butoxyethanol, a solvent absorbed through the skin that irritates eyes and may damage red blood cells. A secret blend of alcohol ethoxylate surfactants; some members of this chemical family are banned in the European Union. This concentrated product is sold in a ready-to-use spray bottle despite instructions to dilute, even for heavy cleaning.

4. Scrubbing Bubbles Antibacterial Bathroom Cleaner & Extend-A-Clean Mega Shower Foamer
These products contain up to 10 percent DEGBE, also called brotherliness, a solvent banned in the European Union at concentrations above 3 percent in aerosol cleaners. It can irritate and inflame the lungs.

5. Dynamo and Fab Ultra liquid laundry detergents
These contain formaldehyde, also known as formalin, classified as a known human carcinogen by the U.S. government and World Health Organization. Formaldehyde can cause asthma and allergies. The company divulges the presence of formaldehyde in the product only on technical disclosures for workers.

Sadly, this is just the tip of the iceberg. See the full sneak-peak here: See EWG's Guide to Healthy Cleaning at http://www.ewg.org/guides/cleaners.[209]

There are many ecological, toxic chemical free cleaners. Brands like Dr. Bronners, Meyers, Biokleen, and Ecover, etc.

Or, make your own cleaners with some of these basic ingredients: Vinegar, baking soda, lemon juice, hydrogen peroxide, washing soda, castile soap, and a few essential oils.

It's very important to make good choices, not only in our food, but anything we drink, breathe, or put on our bodies. All our choices affect our health, for the better or for the worse. I'm not sure about you, but to me, there is no price tag too great for good health. Luckily, it's not a literal price tag but the price of effort, education, standing up for and doing what's best for you and your family.

CHAPTER 87

DRY SKIN BRUSHING

I LOVE BRUSHING my skin. Not only is it good for you, but it feels great. I must admit that I'm much better at it during the summer months, when it's warm and I don't mind standing in the shower brushing my skin before turning the shower on. In the winter months I'm wimpy about the cold, and can't stand more than 30 seconds without the hot water on me! Why brush your skin? And what does that even mean?

What if I told you there's a simple wellness trick that only takes five minutes a day, costs nothing, and helps to cleanse your body, inside and out? Dry skin brushing has a number of health benefits and is so simple to do.

So how does it work?
Your skin, the largest organ in the human body, is an organ of elimination. One third of your body's toxins are excreted through the skin, and dry brushing helps to unclog your pores and excrete toxins that have become trapped in the skin.

To get started, follow the simple steps below.

1. Purchase a natural (not synthetic) bristle brush with a long handle so you can reach all areas of your body.
2. Get naked, and stand in a bathtub or on a tiled surface to catch the falling skin. (It's a bit gross, I know.)
3. Begin brushing by starting at your feet and moving in long sweeping motions toward your heart. Always brush toward your heart.
4. Brush each area several times, overlapping as you go.

5. Take care as you brush over more sensitive areas, such as your breasts. Your skin will become less sensitive the more you dry brush.
6. Once you've brushed your entire body, jump in the shower. (I like to alternate between the hottest water temperature I can tolerate and the coldest. This stimulates blood circulation, bringing more blood to the top layers of the skin.)
7. After getting out of the shower, pat your skin dry and apply a natural fruit oil like rose hip or coconut oil.
8. Continue to dry brush your entire body every day; twice a day is recommended for the best results. Remember to clean your brush with soap and water once a week. Leave it to dry in a clean, sunny spot to avoid any mildew accumulation on your brush.

Try this for 30 days and see the results for yourself!

Some benefits of dry skin brushing:

1. **You'll exfoliate dead skin.**
   Forget your in-shower loofah and body scrubs, brushing will ensure that you have silky-smooth skin all year!
2. **It stimulates your lymphatic system.**
   Dry brushing your skin will kick-start your lymphatic system, which helps you to remove toxins from your body. The stiffer the bristles on the brush, the more lymphatic stimulation you'll create.
3. **Dry brushing helps to reduce cellulite.**
   Cellulite is simply toxic materials that have accumulated in your body's fat cells and are trapped, unable to be eliminated from the body. Forget about liposuction; dry skin brushing helps to break down any trapped toxins within the body and help your body to eliminate them through its usual elimination channels.
4. **It unclogs pores.**
   Dry skin brushing unclogs your skin's pores and helps your skin absorb more nutrients. Daily skin brushing promotes healthy, breathing skin. It's a real treat for the largest organ in our bodies![210]

CHAPTER 88

EXERCISE

I GREW UP watching my mom do aerobics to Joanie Greggains' videos[211] *Your Heart Says Thank You*, and my dad lifting weights in the garage, listening to John Denver records, "country road, take me home, sing it with me…to the place, I belong, West Virginia, mountain mama, take me home, country road." Sorry for the detour. That song makes me happy! Later, my parents got into swimming and would go to the YMCA and swim laps.

As for me, in high school I played basketball, ran track and marched in the band. I did not really do any exercise outside of school. When my husband and I first got married, my mom gave us her Joanie Greggains' tapes and I continued the aerobics tradition. I did not really start exercising seriously until after our second daughter was born, when my size 8 jeans went to a 12 and my weight was not coming back down. To try to get my weight down I did the *Body for Life*[212] diet. In this diet they recommend rotating cardio exercise with weight lifting. As poor newlyweds we found a free weight bench at the side of the road and bought a $25 exercise bike out of the penny saver, which I'm proud to report I put 5000 miles on before our teething toddler ate the tension knob off the bike; that can't be healthy! After 12 weeks I had lost 20 pounds and felt great, which is why I stayed on that diet and exercise plan for 10 more years.

After that, a friend of mine introduced me to Zumba. Boy was that fun; awkward, but fun! I love a good beat and while I can't bust a move on my own too well, I can copy a dance and look only halfway dorky while doing it. I also loved the weight and aerobic classes and the stair climber had to be my favorite. Not sure why, but I got a thrill from watching sweat bead up on the back on my hands and roll off. I knew I was working hard when that happened!

Years later, I noticed a super fit mom bringing her daughter to the same preschool that my son attended. This mom would show up in exercise clothes, and she had such a lean and strong body. I wanted to know what she was doing. I asked her, and she told me her name was Kelli Russell and that she is a yoga teacher. I thought, "oh no, there is no way I'm doing yoga! I tried it once and it was the most boring thing I have ever done in my life!"

The next Friday I was waiting in line at the gym for my Zumba® class. We were waiting because there was a room full of "sleeping yoga" students doing who knows what. When their class ended, they came out looking all slim and toned, and guess who their teacher was? Kelli Russell! We said "hi" and she invited me to come to her class again. I probably said, "yeah, I should come sometime." I was thinking that there was no way I'd go to her class! But five days a week I'd see her at the preschool looking how I wanted to look; and every Friday night I'd see her and all her fit class "sleeping" before Zumba®, and I wanted to know the secret. I was also really intrigued with her as a person and wanted to get to know her better. I thought I would like to be her friend. I decided to do the unthinkable and take her yoga class!

Wow, what an adventure Kelli's yoga class was! First of all it was nothing like the first yoga class I had taken that bored me out of my mind. I could not believe how hard Kelli's class was, and I really could not believe how sore I was for about five days after her class! I was a gym rat working out every day, yet I got totally beat up by her yoga class. And, did I say that I LOVED it? I loved Kelli as a teacher too. I was hooked. I found out about that sleeping thing they do; it's called shavasana. It's a resting pose, and is the final pose of the class. I had missed all the crazy, hard, and fun poses they were doing for 50 minutes before I got in line for Zumba®, and only watched them "sleep." I spent the next few years taking Kelli's yoga classes until breaking my back detoured me from her classes for almost 3 years! I am so happy to be back to yoga with the amazing Kelli Russell!

Exercise is healthy for so many reasons, and I'm sure that you're already aware of them. For me, one of the most important things exercise gave me was a stress outlet. As most people do in this modern age, I had taken on a lot in my life; my husband, four kids, a real estate business and service in my church and community. I was really not taking much time for myself. It's kind of odd, but I never really had any hobbies until the last few years. I liked to work, and work was not only my job but my hobby. That led to lots of long hours and late nights, and I really needed a stress outlet. Exercise was perfect for helping me to unwind. Yoga especially taught me to calm down and slow down. It took something much more traumatic however to teach me to slow down in my life, not just on my yoga mat. That something was a broken back. Too bad I didn't completely learn my lesson in yoga! There's a hint for the rest of you.

On August 10, 2013, I broke my back and tore a ligament in my hip in a hiking accident. By December 2013, I tried to go back to yoga but by February 2014 I had to stop because of hip and back pain. In May 2015 I had back surgery, as none of the alternative methods of healing were helping with my pain, at least not enough to get me off pain killers, and I wanted my life back. Doctors inserted rods and screws and a synthetic disk in my back in an attempt to reduce the pain. Unfortunately, the surgery didn't fix the pain. Pain is hard, pain hurts, pain is sad, frustrating and debilitating. Pain is also change, learning, growth and knowledge. For almost three years I did my best every day to lean into the good and try to not let the pain drag me down as it so easily can. So many people asked me how I was doing, accepting my new life of pain? Many people told me that once you have a bad back it's never the same, and they felt so bad for me because I was so young. I knew this pain would pass; I could not live like this, and I'd search for an answer until I found one.

There was a silver lining, however. During my years of severe pain, I can honestly say that I have never been happier, which is quite interesting to me because it's kind of hard to be happy while feeling chronic and debilitating pain. There is so much good in my life that the sun hides the shadows (most of the time)! There is so much I am grateful for. There is so much I am learning, and waking up to know. I feel enlightened every day. I am so grateful for my family, friends, and religion; for God who knows me and loves me perfectly and incomprehensibly and lightened my burdens to make them bearable. Lying in bed, I had lots of time to appreciate the things that I was too busy to notice before. Now that my back is better, life is much more fun! However, I can look back and see how I was strengthened at the time to endure and learn what I needed to.

I finally made it back to yoga in March 2016, and boy, was that a happy day! Whatever type of exercise you choose, just do it! It's great for your brain, heart, bones, and muscles. Exercise also removes toxins from your system and makes you feel great. Don't overdo it. Don't hurt yourself. Be sensible, and remember that you only have one body; so learn from me, and don't carelessly hurt it because the price is too high.

CHAPTER 89

MOBILITY

REMEMBER THAT AWESOME and amazing Kelli Russell I keep mentioning? Check out this article she wrote on mobility.

If you don't move it, you'll lose it! And you don't want to lose it! To maintain or increase joint mobility, create some space for blood, nutrients, and energy to flow through, and find a greater sense of ease in your body, begin each morning with these 10 movements, and your joints will LOVE you!

Begin Standing Up

1. **Ankle circles.** *Hands on hips, extend your right leg out to the side and point your toe, roll your ankle in circles clockwise, then counter-clockwise about 5x each direction. Repeat with left ankle.*
2. **Knee Pumps.** *With knees together, bend your knees and place your hands on your knees. Roll your knees 5x to the right, 5x to the left.*
3. **Pelvic Rolls** – *Feet hips width, hands on hips. Move hips around in big circles (like hula hooping). 5x to the right, 5x to the left.*
4. **Trunk Twists** – *Feet a bit wider than hips width apart, knees slightly bent. Twist your torso as you swing your arms side to side.*
5. **Wrist Rolls** – *Interlace fingers, elbows together at heart height. Make figure 8s going one direction a few times, then switch direction of rotation.*
6. **Shoulder Rolls** – *arms relaxed by sides, roll shoulders in a circle: up, forward then down 3x. Switch, roll shoulders up back and down a few times.*

7. **Neck Circles** – Roll neck around in circles clockwise 5x, counterclockwise 5x.
8. **Head Realign/Shoulder blade Stretch** – place fingertips on outer ears, elbows out wide. Touch elbows together (or as close as you can get them) keeping head in line with shoulders, then draw elbows out again. 5x
9. **Spinal Roll.** Legs a bit wider than hips width apart in Open Horse Stance (Separate your feet wider than hips-width apart, toes out, heels in. Bend your knees as close to 90° as you can without strain, bringing your knees directly over your ankles. Make sure that your knees are pointing the same direction as your toes.) Place hands on knees, undulate your spine in a wavelike motion, beginning with your tailbone and extending up the spine. 5x
10. **Uddiyana Bandha** – Remain in Open Horse Stance with hands on knees. Inhale through your nose, exhale through your nose. Contract your abdominal muscles to press out as much air as possible, then relax your abdominals. Dr.aw your chin to your chest and take a "mock inhale" -expand your ribs as if you're going to inhale, but instead of actually inhaling, suck your abdominal muscles up, underneath your ribcage, hollowing out your belly. Attempt to hold for 15 seconds, then inhale slowly. Take a few regular breaths between each Uddiyana Bandha, repeat 3x. (This energy lock helps draw your pelvis away from your hip joint, creating space there).[213]

CHAPTER 90

POP!

A FEW YEARS back I was doing some political work, and in talking to parents I was so surprised to hear many of them say that they believe one way but their kids believed another. The parents conveyed that they wanted to let their kids find their own way. I was really surprised. Why are parents not teaching their children what they know and believe? I think some parents try to be too open minded and don't guide their kids in the name of acceptance or open mindedness. Some parents might be too busy trying to be a friend instead of a parent. I'm not saying force your kids to think how and what you think, but at least give it your best effort in areas that you feel strongly about. When you don't teach your children, it's like sending them down a whitewater rapid without a guide and thinking you are doing them a favor. Save your children from learning life's lessons the hard way. Open your mouth. Stand up for what you know to be true. I heard a speaker at a women's conference that said we need to be like a popcorn kernel. We need to pop (speak up) when something is being said that we feel the need to stand up for. Don't be shy, that's the time to pop! Not in an aggressive manner, no exploding, just share what you know to be true. Don't hold it in.

Regarding food choices, you have countless opportunities to teach your children by word of mouth and by your example. Don't eat junk food and expect them to eat healthfully. Don't eat healthy yourself and let them eat junk without caring. I realize you can't, and should not, force them to follow your advice; but do work hard to teach them the "why" of plant based eating and hopefully they will make healthy choices on their own. My kids have all followed my health advice to different degrees. I am grateful that they think about their food choices, and how it affects them and our planet and the animals. Healthy food choices are life and death for our bodies and our planet. This topic is worth popping over! "It takes Nothing to join the crowd. It takes Everything to stand alone.[214]" You can do it!

When we first changed our eating habits, there was a lot of complaining around our house. My husband reminded me that changing our diet was like turning a cruise ship around. They don't turn on a dime. With love and patience, I got the ship turned around, mostly!

Don't think for a minute that I've got my family eating perfectly. They eat healthy at home and I encourage them to make those same choices away from home too. I don't want to force them to eat healthy. I want to teach them why to eat healthy, and I hope that they decide to stick to it when mom isn't watching. I realize as a kid it might be harder to make this kind of a decision when it might be harder to grasp the consequences of taking the "I don't care" approach. No matter what they choose. I love them. That's my most important job!

CHAPTER 91

NATURAL PEST CONTROL

MARYANN SAWYER'S BLOG has some really helpful tips for natural pest control.

...the BEST way to control pests is to not invite them inside in the first place. Most bugs are attracted to food and water, so keeping your kitchen clean, taking out the garbage regularly, and storing food and drinks in tight containers will deter most insects, and other pests. Removing water sources will also go a long way towards solving your bug problem, as will sealing off their point of entry.

If these methods don't take care of the problem though here are 31 MORE all-natural remedies for those critters that are really BUGGING you!

The pest I have had the most questions/concerns raised about is ANTS! For being such a tiny little thing, ants sure can be a nuisance! Here are some tips to keep them out of your house and away from your picnics.

ANTS

Keep It Clean, Folks!
Keep your kitchen counters free of crumbs and sticky spots, cover the sugar and the honey jar. Wiping down surfaces can go a long way toward keeping your home pest free!

Cucumber
Set out cucumber peels or slices in the kitchen or at the ants' point of entry. Many ants have a natural aversion to cucumber.

Mint
Leave a few tea bags of mint tea near areas where the ants seem most active.

Block The Entry
Trace the ant column back to their point of entry. Set any of the following items at the entry area in a small line, which ants will not cross: cayenne pepper, citrus oil (can be soaked into a piece of string), lemon juice, cinnamon or coffee grounds.

Light It Up
Leave a small night light on for a few nights in the area with the most ant activity. The change in light can disrupt and discourage their foraging patterns.

Build A Moat
If ants are attacking your pets' food bowls, clean the floor thoroughly with hot, soapy water to eliminate the ants' trail, then keep them from finding the food dish again by placing the food bowl into a shallow pan of soapy water.

Diatomaceous Earth
Diatomatious earth (often referred to as "DE") is a talc-like powder that is the fossilized remains of marine phytoplankton. When sprinkled on bugs the fine powder absorbs lipids from the waxy outer layer of the insects' exoskeletons, causing them to dehydrate.

Cornmeal
Put small piles of cornmeal where you see ants. They eat it, take back to their home, can't digest it, and expire. It may take a week or so, especially if it rains, but it works and you don't have the worry about pets or small children being harmed.

Homemade Ant Bait
Dissolve 1 teaspoon of boric acid and 6 tablespoons of sugar in 2 cups of water. Soak cotton balls in this bait solution. (Boric acid is a low-toxicity mineral, but do keep it away from children and pets because it can cause skin, mouth, stomach, and eye irritation.)

Place one or two cotton balls on an inverted jar lid and saturate with the mixture.

Place the jar lids along ant trails, or where ants have been seen.

Replenish the liquid as it dries until the ants are gone.

Be patient! The key is to get worker ants to continually carry low doses of boric acid back to feed the ants in their nest.

Cover Their Trail

Ants leave a scented trail so other ants can find their way to food. Routinely wash away these invisible trails with a vinegar-based cleanser made from 1?4 cup vinegar, 2 cups water and 10 to 15 drops of peppermint, clove, eucalyptus or melaleuca essential oil.

MOSQUITOES

Block Them

Mosquitos are most active in the early morning and early evening. They seek areas of still air because they are hampered by breezes. Close windows and doors on the side of your house which are opposite the breeze.

Remove Water

The most important measure you can take is to remove standing water sources. Change birdbaths, wading pools and your pet's water bowl twice a week. Keep your house gutters clean and well-draining. Remove yard items that collect water.

BBQ Helper

If you're using the barbeque, throw a bit of sage or rosemary on the coals to repel mosquitoes.

Garlic

An effective natural bug repellent, mix one part garlic juice with five parts of water in a small spray bottle. Shake well before using. Spray lightly on exposed body parts for an effective repellent lasting five to six hours. Strips of cotton cloth can also be dipped in this mixture and hung in areas such as patios, as a localized deterrent.

Build A Bat House
Some bat species can eat up to 1,000 mosquitoes in an hour! You can attract these beneficial bug eaters by installing a bat house in your yard.

Neem Oil
Neem oil is a natural vegetable oil extracted from the Neem tree in India. The leaves, seeds and seed oil of the neem tree contain sallanin, a compound which has effective mosquito repelling properties. Neem oil is a natural product and is safe to use. Just add a few drops of oil to your favorite lotion and apply the mixture to your body.

Plant More Flowers
Plant some catnip (Nepeta cataria) in your garden; not only will it repel mosquitoes, but you'll get some pretty flowers, too. Other mosquito-repelling plants include rosemary, marigolds, citronella grass, and lemon balm.

Light A Candle
Make your own mosquito-repelling candles using a mixture of essential oils and melted wax. A good rule of thumb is to use about 1/2 ounce to 1 ounce of essential oil per pound of wax.

Here are some good mosquito-repelling essential oil blends to add to your candles from from about.com.

Recipe #1 – Simple and Spicy
5 parts Citronella
5 parts Lavender
5 parts Clove

Recipe #2 – Bright and Energetic
5 parts Citronella
5 parts Lavender
5 parts Peppermint

Recipe #3 – Deep and Green
10 parts Citronella
10 parts Cedarwood
5 parts Eucalyptus
5 parts Rosemary

DIY Mosquito Repellant Mixture
For a do-it-yourself mosquito repellent, you'll need essential oil and something to mix it with, like vodka, olive oil, or witch hazel. For best results, combine a few different essential oils such as lemon, eucalyptus, citronella, cinnamon, cedarwood, and juniper berry.

Cover Up
Common sense is as good a guide as any. To avoid getting bitten by mosquitoes, wear long pants and long sleeved shirts, and a hat or scarf. Use window and door screens and put mosquito netting over infant carriages or strollers.

Bug-Off Drink
Nutritionally, you can drink a tablespoon or two of organic apple cider vinegar and eat lots of garlic. Vitamin B1 taken daily is also supposed to help repel insects.

FLIES

Herbal Sachets
Place sachets made from small squares of cheesecloth and filled with crushed mint, bay leaves, cloves or eucalyptus around the house to repel flies.

DIY Flypaper
Mix 1/4 cup corn syrup, 1 tablespoon granulated sugar and 1 tablespoon brown sugar in a small bowl. Cut strips of brown kraft paper and soak them in the sugar mixture. Let them dry overnight. To hang, poke a small hole at the top of each strip and hang with string.

Sweet Basil
Plant sweet basil next to the doors, or plant it in containers. The flies will stay far away. Cut a nice size bunch of it to take with you when you go on picnics. As an added bonus, mosquitoes don't like it either.

Eucalyptus Oil
For creating an area that's free of flies, apply eucalyptus essential oil to a small cloth or rag and leave it out.

SPIDERS

Spiders Hate Peppermint
Place a few drops of peppermint essential oil into a spray bottle. Add a squirt of liquid detergent and fill the bottle with water. Spray the mixture on cobwebs, around doors and windows, around the lawn and garden and on any surfaces where spiders lurk. In addition to having a pleasant aroma, this mixture is nontoxic and safe to use around children and pets.

Coconut Oil And Vinegar
The combination of coconut oil and white vinegar also makes an effective spray for repelling spiders. As oils may stain or cause spots, test the mixture on a small, hidden area of carpets, curtains or upholstered furniture.

Citrus Essential Oils
Spiders taste through their feet, and in addition to peppermint they do not like the taste of citrus which includes lemon, lime, tangerine, and wild orange. Although it will not kill them, it will make them avoid places where they can "taste" them. Always purchase real essential oils and not synthetic versions.

Eliminate Hiding Places
Spiders thrive in dark, cluttered places, so keep stacks of debris, woodpiles and thick plant growth away from the sides of the house. The fewer places spiders can easily inhabit, the more effectively they can be repelled.

Seal It Up
Seal cracks in the foundation and close gaps in windows or beneath doorways to deny spiders access to the premises.

And last but not least .an all natural, homemade insect repellent that should help out with all of the above!

ALL PURPOSE, ALL NATURAL BUG SPRAY

Homemade Insect Repellent Recipe

- *8 oz apple cider vinegar, witch hazel, or vodka*
- *45 drops peppermint essential oil*
- *15 drops lemon or wild orange essential oil*

Mix ingredients in a spray bottle and apply liberally. Store in the fridge when not in use. Should last 2-3 months[215].

CHAPTER 92

SUNSHINE

THERE ARE SO many reasons to get out in the sunshine. Let's start with vitamin D, which your body makes from the sun's rays. I've read that noon time sun is best for vitamin D absorption and you need about 5-15 minutes without sunscreen on your arms, hands and face three times per week. Take time to get your vitamin D while enjoying those wonderful warm sun rays! Some people say to take a vitamin D supplement, but supplements don't give you all the same benefits as the sun. It's like taking vitamin C instead of eating an orange. Our bodies are made to eat whole foods and function best when we do. Not even scientists can explain the complex metabolic reactions that happen when you eat one plant food item. Don't miss out by taking supplements instead. Of course the vitamin companies tell you it's just as good as the sun, but remember they are making money from the sales.

The sun has many more benefits that just the Vitamin D.

A few known benefits of sunshine:
Lowers cholesterol, lowers blood pressure, promotes thyroid stimulation, regulates the immune system, stimulates insulin production, Improves heart muscle contractility.

Currently prescribed for the treatment of:
Rickets, osteomalacia, osteoporosis, acne, eczema, psoriasis, neonatal jaundice, and depression.

Has a role in the prevention of:
Osteoporosis, heart disease, type-1 diabetes, multiple sclerosis, rheumatoid arthritis, Crohn's disease, and cancers of the prostate, breast, colon, lung, ovary, bladder, uterus, esophagus, stomach, pancreas, kidney, multiple myeloma and non-Hodgkin's lymphoma[216].

One of my favorite places to enjoy the sun is in my garden. Not only am I getting all the benefits listed above, I'm growing wonderfully delicious and nutritious food to add to my health and the health of my family.

CHAPTER 93

SLEEP

It's 11:18 p.m. on a Friday night, after a long week; and since I want to be a good example, and don't want to stay up late typing a lecture to you about how you need to sleep more, I think this is a very good place to stop and continue on in the morning.

And it's another Friday night, now 12:25 a.m.—time to stop typing. Glad I get to sleep in tomorrow. I really need to work on getting more sleep! How does that saying go? Early to bed, early to rise, makes a man healthy, wealthy and wise. I am working on this sleeping thing. I'm getting better!

Great reasons to sleep longer:

- *Improved memory*
- *Live Longer*
- *Reduced Inflammation*
- *Spur Creativity*
- *Better Athlete*
- *Better Grades*
- *Better Attention*
- *Healthier Body Weight*
- *Less Stress*
- *Avoid Depression*
- *Avoid Accidents*[217]

I might add, getting enough sleep helps you avoid that miserable feeling of your eyelids closing and just wishing you could go to sleep right then but it's the middle of the day and you can't! Let's get more sleep! Sweet dreams.

CHAPTER 94

FIND A HOBBY

WHERE IS THE joy? What do I like to do? What do your kids like to do? I used to ask myself these questions, and I think the main reason was because I didn't take time to explore any hobbies. I worked really hard taking care of my family, in my real estate career, in church and community service, and exercising. Those, although enjoyable, were really not hobbies. As the years go on, I have found hobbies that I never knew I'd be interested in.

I now love gardening, cooking, creating recipes, writing, speaking, and learning about health and healing; and I'm even starting to learn the fine art of relaxing! I am also working on not judging myself by what I do but by who I am. It's really nice to "be" instead of "do." I've been forced to learn this lesson with my past health challenges. I guess a broken back was what I needed to learn some hard life lessons. Too bad I was not open minded enough to learn the easy way. Find a new hobby and pursue it with a passion! No excuses!

Check out the story of Dr. Weiss who decided to change what his life looked like. I love stories like these! Help your kids find their passions too!

Meet the Physician-Farmer Who Grows The Plants He Prescribes To His Patients[218]
In 2012, Dr. Ron Weiss cashed in most of his assets to buy a 342-acre farm—a National Historic Landmark—in bucolic Long Valley, N.J., which is an hour west of Manhattan, N.Y. What inspired an urban primary care doctor who had a thriving practice to take up farming? To find out, we talked to Weiss,

assistant professor of clinical medicine at New Jersey Medical School and the founder of Ethos Health, the first working farm-based medical practice in the country.

Weiss grew up in the 1960s in New Jersey and remembers the farms he visited every season to buy the state's famous peaches, blueberries, and tomatoes. He also remembers how slowly, but surely, the farms started disappearing. As a child, Weiss loved nature, science, and the outdoors. He also dreamed of having a farm of his own one day in his beloved garden state.

As an undergraduate at Rutgers University, he chose to major in botany and also pursued pre-med and piano performance studies. He completed his residency at George Washington University and started working as an emergency room doctor at Cedars-Sinai Medical Center in Los Angeles. It was there that Weiss received the call that would direct the course of his life. "I got the news that my father was diagnosed with pancreatic cancer and was given one month to live," he said. "The cancer had spread to his other organs, so his doctor told him that chemotherapy had little to no chance of shrinking his tumors. So he opted out of treatment and went home to prepare to die. I quit my job in California and returned home to be with him."

This was way before internet research was easy and accessible, so once he got home, Weiss went to the local library in Fair Lawn, N.J., to research alternative treatments to help his father. Weiss had one advantage—his botany training. He explained, "I was always studying the resilience of plants and their ability, given optimal circumstances, to fend off their own diseases." Since over one-third of all pharmaceuticals are derived from plants, Weiss was always interested in how the full power of plants, rather than extractions, could reverse and prevent illness. "I was distraught and motivated, and I read everything I could get my hands on," he recalled. "I then stumbled upon some first-person stories about how people had found success using a macrobiotic diet as an alternative and complementary cancer treatment."

Witnessing Firsthand the Power of a Plant-Based Diet

He put his father on the macrobiotic diet promoted by Michio Kushi, a leader in the macrobiotic community and food-health movement. It was a plant-based *diet with a focus on grains and vegetables. Dr. Weiss still talks about what happened with amazement:*

"A plant-based diet doesn't sound strange now, but it was shocking to people at that time. This was in 1991. On this diet, my father lived for 18 more months. He didn't just survive, limping along—he rapidly improved and soon felt better than he had for most of his adult life. His severe abdominal pains vanished and a week later he was able to return to his work as an attorney. In another week he was back in the gym, and then started running every day. It was incredible. His doctors were shocked by his CT scans—he had a 50 percent reduction in tumor masses.

"That's when I realized that the connection between food and health was so powerful, and that I wanted to do work that incorporated the healing power of good food. After my father died, I went back to work as an ER doctor and eventually set up a primary and multi-specialty busy practice in West New York, N.J. Plant-based nutrition was the foundation of my daily practice, but I knew that I eventually wanted to incorporate it into a broader lifestyle approach and get patients invested in how their food is grown."

After 16 years, Weiss realized it was time to break free from the more traditional setting and create a new paradigm in medical care. "I envisioned a different type of health care—one that reveals to people the root causes [of] their suffering and strives to remove them." He spent five years looking for the right farm, sold most of his assets—including his medical practice—and convinced his wife and children to go all-in on the dream of Ethos Health. It's been a bumpy but exciting road for Weiss and his family with all the rigors of relocation, start-up struggles, running a working farm, and creating a new life from scratch. It's hard to be the first.

CHAPTER 95

NO MAMMOGRAMS!

Every time you get a mammogram you increase your chances of getting breast cancer, because of the cell mutating properties of mammography. Share this information with your grown up kids! Mammograms are not a good means of early detection; mammograms only find 52% of cancers. If you have a lump, you need to get an ultrasound, which does not have any cell mutating properties. If you are interested in early detection a thermogram is what you want. Thermography senses heat and can find cancer cells without causing further damage to your body.[219]

With cancer, it's important to fight against the cause! I believe the cause is our food. When people change how they eat, they change their health almost immediately. They still live in a polluted world, they still have "bad genes" or disease that "runs in the family," but they heal themselves and prevent disease with a change in diet even with all other factors remaining the same.

Cancer doubles every100 days on average. If you are eating a whole food, plant based low fat diet, you can slow that progress and some say even stop the cancer. In other words, we know the cause and we can stop fueling the fire! Why won't we, as Americans, make a huge course correction? It's because we choose not to, purely and simply. Maybe we don't believe it. Maybe we don't want to believe it. Change is hard; but so is chemo, surgery, radiation, losing your hair, having low immunity, feeling sick, fatigued and even dying.

In Dr. McDougall's August 2014 Newsletter,[220] he shares his take on early detection, which he does not recommend. He does not even recommend thermogrophy. Read his newsletter regarding not only mammograms, but all early detection methods and what is recommended not only by him but also by the US Preventative Task Force (USPSTF.)[221]

"*Created in 1984, the U.S. Preventive Services Task Force is an independent, volunteer panel of national experts in prevention and evidence-based medicine. The Task Force works to improve the health of all Americans by making evidence-based recommendations[222] about clinical preventive services such as screenings, counseling services, and preventive medications. All recommendations are published on the Task Force's website and/or in a peer-reviewed journal and the Cochrane Collaboration[223]*."

"*We are a global independent network of researchers, professionals, patients, carers, and people interested in health. Cochrane contributors- 37,000 from more than 130 countries - work together to produce credible, accessible health information that is free from commercial sponsorship and other conflicts of interest. Many of our contributors are world leaders in their fields - medicine, health policy, research methodology, or consumer advocacy - and our groups are situated in some of the world's most respected academic and medical institutions. Our work is recognized as representing an international gold standard for high quality, trusted information.[224]*"

Dr. McDougall says, "women often ask me how they should explain to their doctor why they do not want a mammogram. *Mammography Screening: Truth, Lies and Controversy*[225] may help. I consider Dr. Gotzsche the world's foremost expert on mammography research. His book is about ethics in medicine and the influence of self-interest, power, and money on scientific publication. Dr. Gotzsche correctly describes many of the people behind current recommendations for mammogram as liars involved in scientific misconduct that has killed and maimed millions of women. His work shows that routine mammograms (1) do not save women's lives, (2) increase the number of women over-diagnosed with cancer (they would never have known they were sick if not for the mammogram testing), and (3) increase a women's chance of having a mastectomy."

Think twice before you agree to any medical testing. If you eat a whole food, plant based diet; you have the least chance of ever developing any modern disease. What an amazing blessing we can take advantage of!

CHAPTER 96

GROW A GARDEN

GARDENING IS FUN and delicious—and organic, I hope. Gardening gets the whole family involved in a great cause. I have so many fun memories of gardens. My family actually has a history of gardens. My mom says that my great grandpa had a garden in Switzerland and people would travel to come and see it. My grandparents had a huge garden and orchard that I remember them working in a lot. My mom cried a lot over her garden as she watched the pests eat it before she could harvest, especially those darn gophers. Poor mom! I've enjoyed planting many gardens with my family. My youngest likes to help me in my garden the most. The best part, besides our quality time together, is that he loves to eat the veggies as we work in the garden together. He especially loves pulling snap peas off the vines and eating them while we work. He also likes to bring his friends through the garden and feed them all his favorites. The strawberries and hula berries (they look like a light pink strawberry with a pineapple strawberry flavor) and tomatoes are my favorite, and the cucumbers too. This year, due to my back injury I've planted a table(s) top container garden which I love to water and trim and eat from every day!

I am so excited about a gardening movie I watched recently called *Back to Eden*.[226] Paul Gautschi wanted a garden but only had a 1/2 gallon per minute well. He prayed to God and asked how he could grow a garden. He learned that God's garden has no irrigation and his didn't need it either. Wait, what did you say? Paul started growing a garden the way plants and trees grown in nature, with a deep covering over the soil, and he has the most amazing garden; and he has not watered it for 31 years! People come from all over to see Paul's garden and to taste his delicious food.

Everywhere in nature the soil is covered, except where man has used it. The cover holds in moisture and builds new soil. Soil is a living organism and it needs to be covered. When the cover comes off, the land is damaged. It takes 100 years to build an inch of top soil. Four tons of soil per acre is what farmers say is okay to lose per year due to winds and runoff. There is a better way. We can't get this wonderful soil back as it grows so slowly. Don't try to change nature; work with it like God does. Check out Paul's website for a quick guide on how to grow your best garden every with no tilling or irrigation![227] http://www.backtoedenfilm.com/how-to-grow-an-organic-garden.html

CHAPTER 97

TO THINE OWN SELF BE TRUE

How many times have you heard someone say, "listen to your body?" If I had a dollar for every time I heard that, I'd be sitting pretty. If I had a dollar for every time I did that, I'd be "empty in my bank account" as Ketut says in *Eat, Pray. Love.*[228] Even though my health story starts with the rock jump, my pain story starts 25 years earlier.

When I hit puberty, I had terrible menstrual cramps. I thought I would die each month. My mom took me to a gynecologist and told me we'd "talk" to him. A pair of rubber gloves later and a death look towards my mom, he said he didn't really know why I was having so much pain and prescribed me some pain killers. I took the painkillers and did my best to survive each month, dazed from the pain killers and with numb legs because that's one thing that would happen to me. I could walk; I just could not feel my legs. I had terrible pain in my low back, hips and lower abdomen. I was a busy, high achieving athletic student. I did not let pain stop me from doing what I wanted to do, like marching in parades as drum major of the band, running sprints, hurdles, relays and jumps for the track team, shooting hoops for the basketball team, get straight A's of course and working in a deli on the weekends to pay for the BMW I bought myself when I was 16 years old. See, I really am a type A! I was in miserable pain but still did what I wanted to do and that pattern continued. I ignored my body and pressed forward.

I met my husband when I was 14. We got engaged when I was 17, and married at 18. Before we had our first baby, when I was 21, we were on a trip and I didn't have my ibuprofen handy (which I had switched to since it didn't have the sleepy effects of the pain killers). Unfortunately, I was taking 30 Ibuprofen per day during that one week each month and really ignoring the warning labels about liver damage, etc. My husband could not believe the pain I was in, and still talks about it to this day. Luckily, someone found me some Ibuprofen and I survived that trip. As I started having children, my pain improved a bit; but once I was finished having children, wow, the pain came back with a vengeance. I was back to taking 30 Ibuprofen per day and going about my busy life of raising four kids, selling real estate, serving in my church and in my community.

One day my stomach decided it had had enough Ibuprofen and it felt like it was on fire. I found out I had ulcers in my stomach and bladder, and according to blood tests I was also in liver failure. I was left to endure the monthly pain because my body couldn't take any more pain killers. I'd sit on the couch for a week each month rocking myself and crying, and when it would end I'd turn back into super woman. By age 34, I could not take it anymore and the doctors did exploratory surgery to see what was going on. They suspected that I had endometriosis; and they did find some and removed it during the surgery. Unfortunately, that surgery did not help my monthly pain. At 35 years old, I had a full hysterectomy and when the surgery pain dissipated, my pain was gone! I had new problems like my skin decided to age 10+ years over the next two years due to the lack of hormones, hot flashes etc., but anything was better than pain.

I thought I'd been through enough pain, but after breaking my back on Aug 10, 2013 and then spending three years recovering, I've learned a lot about listening to my body. When I move, stand, sit or walk I try to pay attention to what my body is doing and change the things that are not right. For example, when I put my mascara on, I lean forward to look into the mirror while standing on my right leg only and learning into the mirror in a weird, unbalanced way. This action is not great for my body so I quit doing it. I had my left foot in an odd position while driving too. Little bad habits can add up. Pay attention to your body. Sit up straight, stand up tall, and walk like an Egyptian. Just kidding! I was making sure my book was not putting you to sleep. Ha!)

Here are some things that helped me get to know myself that I would also recommend to you:

Get on a treadmill with no TV and no music and walk. What can you learn? When I did this I felt like there was too much tension in my hips. The action of my walk was starting in my hips and they were pushing my legs forward and flopping my feet down with a smack. It was subtle but obvious when I paid attention. Why was I walking like this? Later, I was watching one of my daughter's walk and she was doing the exact same thing I was. I guess I modeled it perfectly wrong for her. Most of us don't know that we are moving in a way that can cause pain down the road, stop and pay attention. It's worth it.

I recommend the book *Full Catastrophe Living*[229] (using the wisdom of your body and mind to face stress, pain and illness) by Jon Kabat-Zinn, Ph.D. He talks about how amazingly connected we are with our outer body but how disconnected we are with what is happening inside our body. He talks about how most people are insecure with some part of their body and they spend their days obsessed with that instead of being connected to their whole body. He talks about how what we think about our body really limits our experiences. These were interesting things to think about for me and they really rang true. Dr. Kabat-Zinn then teaches you how to get in touch with your whole body. Of course we think we are too busy to buy the book and learn the technique and we are definitely too busy to practice what he teaches but maybe that same thinking is what got us into some of the stress or pain we deal with today. We all have the same 24 hours per day. We don't have a time problem we have a priority problem. Spend some time connecting with your whole body each day.

I'd be remiss if I didn't say to spend some time with your spirit each day too. Our body and spirit are two separate but totally connected entities. A funny story—well, sad, but funny. My mom's mom, grandma Esther passed away and we were at her funeral. My kids were looking at her body lying in the coffin, and my mom said, "it's just like a banana peel. What you see is grandma's peel and her spirit is the banana that is now in heaven." I always thought of it more as a hand in a glove but I guess the banana and peel are the same analogy. My kids looked at me a bit funny, but they knew and understood what she was telling them. Your spirit needs food as much as your body needs food. The difference is that your spirit is quiet and your body is loud. You can go through your whole life and never hear from your spirit if you don't learn how to tune in and listen. Find ways to strengthen your spirit. For me it's daily prayer and scripture study and attending church.

Next, don't' go to the doctor and say, "something is wrong with me and I don't know what." No one is as much of an expert on your body as you are. Spend the time, do the research, find answers and then run them by your doctor. Don't let them guess while you don't even pay attention. There is so much information on the Internet. Take full advantage of it and save yourself from being treated for the wrong condition due to your lack of self-understanding.

Don't overdo it. If your body hurts, it's your biofeedback system trying to tell you something. Pull back. Put your feet up. Take a breather. I learned this lesson the hard way and I hope you can learn from me on this one. My first bad exercise injury was while at yoga class doing a trick I was not ready to do. It took a lot of strength and a lot of flexibility. I had the strength but not the flexibility. So in typical Jenny fashion, I did the pose anyway. Bad decision! Probably four seconds of thinking I was cool and now, years later, I still have a hard time sitting Indian style because of that hip I twisted. I heard my daughter's cross country coach telling one of the kids to take some time off to let their injury heal. Of course the kid didn't want to and coach was forcing him to and the kid was mad. I hope that young man realizes the wisdom and is grateful someday for the pain and suffering that coach saved him and maybe even a long term injury was prevented.

The mind is our next stop. I spent a lot of time seeing doctors trying to get my back to heal. Holistic doctors, medical doctors, surgeons, pain doctors, etc. I begged and pleaded with God to help me find the right person who could help me. After years of searching, I finally met him. A wonderful 87-year-old medical doctor turned kinesiologist. This would be the third kinesiologist I had seen about my back, and I was losing hope that this was the right modality for me. I was praying that this would be the person who could relieve my suffering but I doubted it after so many failed attempts at pain relief. Some people recommended that I just accept the fact that I'd always be in pain. I just couldn't do that. I wanted my life back and was prepared to search and go into debt even until I found a cure.

I was referred to Dr. Jacobs. He asked me why I was there and I told him I wanted to sit in a chair, I wanted to get rid of the excruciating pain, sit in a car, sit at church, exercise, go places with my family, have a social life, get off prescription painkillers. And then the work began! Dr. Jacobs started testing my body via muscle testing asking my subconscious what the issue was. He quickly told me all my pain was emotional not physical. Wait, what? How could that be? I'm a pretty mellow person with a pretty good life. I didn't have any issues, except X, Y, Z of course, but doesn't everyone have a few things? I don't see anyone but me standing in the back of rooms because they can't sit. Any movement aggravates my back, so how could the pain be emotional pain showing up as physical pain? That did not make sense to me. Dr. Jacobs informed me that a lot of things don't make sense but that doesn't mean it's not true. Just look at nature. It's so amazingly complex but just because we don't understand it all, does not mean it doesn't work. I told him I was desperate for relief and was willing to try his method out which was mostly talking!

Many visits later, I was at home standing at my desk working (because it hurts to sit, of course) and my back pain that felt like flames shut off. It just stopped! Like when you turn a light switch from on to off. The pain turned off. I freaked out with excitement and yelled for my husband and kids and told them the thrilling news! After that day the pain would come and go. It never returned with a vengeance like the original pain but felt more like cramping and tight muscles. I worked to continue to learn how to shut that pain off. I learned what thoughts were causing the pain and tried to change my ways to keep that tension away from me. I started sitting, having a social life, got off painkillers and even went back to yoga. What an enormous blessing, and what an odd and shocking way to get it!

With a little bit of coaxing from Dr. Jacobs, I decided it would be nice to learn his methods and use them with my family to help everyone feel their best. Once I learned some of the techniques, I started practicing with friends and family and loved it. I still felt like something was missing however. I kept looking for modalities that could stop the tug of war I felt going on inside me so often. I knew my issues but didn't know how to fix them.

I heard about a method which is a quick and easy way to change the subconscious programs that were running in ways that were not serving me and rewrite the code in my mind so to speak. I tried it! It worked! When my subconscious beliefs changed, so did my happiness, health, relationships, peace and joy. I no longer felt that I was working against myself. I am now thrilled to have a business helping others remove the road blocks keeping them from their best life. I feel so blessed to have a way to help others in any area of their life that they struggle with from pain to relationships to health and prosperity. If you'd like to learn more about this method of change, visit me at www.BalancedYou.org.[230]

For communication with others, a really great book I've recently read is *Feeling Good Together*[231] by David D. Burns, M.D. Dr. Jacobs had been teaching me better communication skills and recommended this book. When you can really understand other people and really be listened to, if feels so good. When you can have a conversation with someone with different views and understand where they are coming from and help them know that you understand without any frustration on either side, it is so rewarding. This is a must read for all married couples and a great read for singles too. I've also listened to this book on Audible[232] which is awesome because I'm always on the go and love to learn as I drive, do dishes, laundry etc.

CHAPTER 98

SKINNY

Do you know anyone who can eat whatever they want and are still skinny? I've never liked those people! I'm sure you can relate to that. I am now grateful, however, that I've always had to fight to keep my weight as it's given me a reason to eat healthy and to exercise. Even though I've always been pretty average, weight wise, I've always had to fight really hard to keep my weight down. It's been so wonderful being on a plant based diet and no longer fighting my weight! It used to be a daily struggle. Notice how many times I used the word fight? I don't even think about it anymore.

I now realize that internal health is much more vital that a couple of extra pounds. Of course they sometimes relate, but plenty of skinny men and women have died of heart disease. Heart disease does not have to be scary even though it's a deadly killer. According to Dr. Esselstyn, heart disease is a toothless paper tiger. What he means by that is it's totally preventable and reversible with the right diet. What a blessing!

In an attempt to keep my weight where I wanted it, I've really been diet obsessed for the past 25 years. When I write all this stuff it sounds quite obsessive; but I guess it was an obsession for me to keep my weight down, and boy, was that a struggle. Here is what I did over the years to get the best shape I could. I play sports in high school, aerobics when I was first got married, used the Body for Life diet after I had my second daughter (and I stuck with that diet for 10 plus years). On this diet, I ate a fist size of carbs and a fist size of protein for six small meals per day, six days a week. Then on my favorite day of the week I could eat what I wanted. I remember cheesecake pastries being on the list! I'd rotate cardio and weights six days per week. I spent all week eating right and exercising and losing weight only to blow it on my "free" day and start all over again. It really felt like Groundhog Day every Monday for 10 years when I'd start the process over! I finally burnt out on that plan and bought into the low carb craze. We started eating tons of chicken and tons of veggies at our house plus lots of protein shakes. I was always a bit uncomfortable with this low carb, high protein diet as it went against my religious eating code. Most members of my church ignored the recommendations of this code anyway, so I justified doing it as well. I mean, if I followed the "make grains your staff of life" recommendation of our church health code, I'd just gain weight (or so I thought), and I was not willing to do that so I stuck with the diet fads of the day. Even on a high protein diet, I still didn't like what my weight was, so I became a calorie counter. I was eating 1600 calories per day when exercising and 1200 calories per day when I was not. The problem was, I could eat 1200 calories pretty quickly during the day, and then what? That is when I invented the After 4 diet. In the After 4 diet, I only ate veggies after 4 p.m. and I didn't count those calories. It was a pretty miserable at dinner time every night, cooking for my family and then watching them eat dinner while I ate raw veggies. My body got used to it after a while, but was this really something that was sustainable or duplicable? Is this how I want to teach my children to eat? No! I didn't know what else to do.

Then I broke my back and really ramped up the calorie counting. I tried my darnedest to only eat 1200 calories, or less, per day since I was moving so much less and didn't want to gain weight as always. To this day, I still find old scratch papers in drawers around the house with my calorie tracking for the day on them. About 17 months after breaking my back, I had a bad allergic reaction to a bone scan injection that almost killed me. That experience got me started on green drinks and eating tons of fruits and veggies. I supplemented my greens with nuts, seeds and oils. I was not eating any high energy food. I'd stuff myself with a ton of fruits and veggies and wash it down with nuts so I didn't starve. I was also cooking my vegetables in oil, and drizzling my salads with oil too. I later learned that oil and nuts are the most calorie dense and fattening food I could be piling onto my fruits and veggies. My body was starving for energy—carbs! I was so full, but so unsatisfied. I was making better food choices, eating for health, but something was missing. I'd cheat to satisfy myself with dark chocolate, but that had to come off my calorie count so I'd eat seven less almonds to make up for the small square of chocolate. Does this sound as ridiculous as it was? Sheesh!

I knew there had to be a better way. I was so tired of obsessing over my weight. I felt that I had to though, because if I slacked off just one or two days, I'd immediately gain weight. I increased my study of The Church of Jesus Christ of Latter-Day Saints' health code, called the *Word of Wisdom*[233], which was written for the entire world, not just members of the Church. I fell in love with the book *Discovering The Word Of Wisdom* by Jane Birch, which gave me a lot of history, background and understanding of this health code. Jane was the first one to tell me that all these oils were not good for me. I didn't believe it! I emailed Jane and asked for confirmation. Did I misunderstand her writings? She quickly and sweetly responded that I had not misunderstood and sent me her Google Docs file with lots of articles about why all oils were bad for me.

In the notes of her book I also found reference to the book *The Starch Solution*[234] by Dr. John McDougall. I read the book along with many others, including *The China Study*[235] and *Prevent and Reverse Heart Disease.*[236] At first I did not agree with *The Starch Solution*. Easting starches went against everything I believed about food and diet because of what I'd been taught/sold by those industries. How can you eat more bread and lose weight? It made no sense! *The Starch Solution* did align with my church health code, however. Could it really be true? I needed to each more starches and that was the secret to health and weight loss? I decided to take a giant leap of faith and tried the starch diet. I started eating grains, beans, corn, potatoes, sweet potatoes with fruit and veggies on the side. I had never felt more full and satisfied. My weight, which was already low from most recently trying to live on green drinks, dropped even more. I stopped weighing myself because my weight was no longer increasing when I didn't keep a close eye on it. I'm so happy to be over this ridiculous weight battle part of my life. I'm even more grateful to have zero worry about developing any modern diseases. I found victory in a whole food, plant based diet!

CHAPTER 99

EMOTIONAL EATING

ALONG WITH THE wrong food choices and sedentary life style of Americans, I think emotional eating is a huge reason for the weight issues of our day. We are so busy doing and trying to keep up with the Jones that we look to all sorts of addictive food for stress management and pleasure. I speak from experience on this topic. I used to have a stash of chocolate in my desk. When I'd get upset, frustrated, stressed or in too much pain, I'd go for the chocolate! The problem is, eating does not help me emotionally feel any better. I'm not eating for hunger or even the love of food. I am not even fully enjoying what I am eating! I'm just stuffing it in my mouth, suppressing my feelings with food.

I decided I'd stop stress eating as much as possible and deal with my feelings in a better way. Part of my dilemma was actually knowing what I was even stress eating about. It turns out that I'm very good at hiding my feelings from myself. I've been working on getting more in touch with what's going on inside me. Instead of eating, I'm doing things like journaling, talking about what might be upsetting me, changing my behavior or attitude, and taking a break and doing something else like playing in my garden.

I also noticed that when Dr. Jacobs helped me to get off pain killers, I started using food to deal with my troubles. The pain killers seemed to numb my pain and also my problems. I guess this might be why it's so hard, besides the physical addiction, for so many people to get off painkillers. I would not have thought of that correlation while

I was taking them, but now, being off them, I can see that to be true for me.

I can see now that eating to numb my pain was the reason I was always fighting my weight. I ate to cover my feelings and those calories on a Standard American Diet really add up. With my diet change, I was now overeating healthy food but I was still really frustrated with myself about this issue. As I mentioned in chapter 97, I learned a method of subconscious belief change which quickly and easily got me past this struggle. Hooray! Actually a hooray does not do the feeling justice. I think I need a hallelujah! If you want to learn more about getting past your emotional eating using the power of the subconscious which is literally 1 million times more powerful than the conscious mind, visit me at www.BalancedYou.org.[237]

More good news, it's pretty hard to gain weight eating starches. It takes your body 30% of the calories eaten in starches to convert that food to use it in your body. Also, starches only have 1 calorie per gram compared with sugars which have 4 calories per gram and fat which has 9 calories per gram. If you are going to overeat, choose starches!

The difference between emotional hunger and physical hunger[238]

Emotional hunger can be powerful. As a result, it's easy to mistake it for physical hunger. But there are clues you can look for that can help you tell physical and emotional hunger apart.

- ***Emotional hunger comes on suddenly.*** *It hits you in an instant and feels overwhelming and urgent. Physical hunger, on the other hand, comes on more gradually. The urge to eat doesn't feel as dire or demand instant satisfaction (unless you haven't eaten for a very long time).*
- ***Emotional hunger craves specific comfort foods.*** *When you're physically hungry, almost anything sounds good—including healthy stuff like vegetables. But emotional hunger craves fatty foods or sugary snacks that provide an instant rush. You feel like you need cheesecake or pizza, and nothing else will do.*

- ***Emotional hunger often leads to mindless eating.*** *Before you know it, you've eaten a whole bag of chips or an entire pint of ice cream without really paying attention or fully enjoying it. When you're eating in response to physical hunger, you're typically more aware of what you're doing.*
- ***Emotional hunger isn't satisfied once you're full.*** *You keep wanting more and more, often eating until you're uncomfortably stuffed. Physical hunger, on the other hand, doesn't need to be stuffed. You feel satisfied when your stomach is full.*
- ***Emotional hunger isn't located in the stomach.*** *Rather than a growling belly or a pang in your stomach, you feel your hunger as a craving you can't get out of your head. You're focused on specific textures, tastes, and smells.*
- ***Emotional hunger often leads to regret, guilt, or shame.*** *When you eat to satisfy physical hunger, you're unlikely to feel guilty or ashamed because you're simply giving your body what it needs. If you feel guilty after you eat, it's likely because you know deep down that you're not eating for nutritional reasons.*

Stop emotional eating tip 1: Identify your triggers
What situations, places, or feelings make you reach for the comfort of food? Most emotional eating is linked to unpleasant feelings, but it can also be triggered by positive emotions, such as rewarding yourself for achieving a goal or celebrating a holiday or happy event. Here are some common causes of emotional eating:

- **Stress** – Ever notice how stress makes you hungry? It's not just in your mind. When stress is chronic, as it so often is in our chaotic, fast-paced world, it leads to high levels of the stress hormone, cortisol. Cortisol triggers cravings for salty, sweet, and high-fat foods—foods that give you a burst of energy and pleasure. The more uncontrolled stress in your life, the more likely you are to turn to food for emotional relief.
- **Stuffing emotions** – Eating can be a way to temporarily silence or "stuff down" uncomfortable emotions, including anger, fear, sadness,

anxiety, loneliness, resentment, and shame. While you're numbing yourself with food, you can avoid the emotions you'd rather not feel.

- **Boredom or feelings of emptiness** – *Do you ever eat simply to give yourself something to do, to relieve boredom, or as a way to fill a void in your life? You feel unfulfilled and empty, and food is a way to occupy your mouth and your time. In the moment, it fills you up and distracts you from underlying feelings of purposelessness and dissatisfaction with your life.*
- **Childhood habits** – *Think back to your childhood memories of food. Did your parents reward good behavior with ice cream, take you out for pizza when you got a good report card, or serve you sweets when you were feeling sad? These emotionally based childhood eating habits often carry over into adulthood. Or perhaps some of your eating is driven by nostalgia—for cherishes memories of grilling burgers in the backyard with your dad, baking and eating cookies with your mom, or gathering around the table with your extended family for a home-cooked pasta dinner.*
- **Social influences** – *Getting together with other people for a meal is a great way to relieve stress, but it can also lead to overeating. It's easy to overindulge simply because the food is there or because everyone else is eating. You may also overeat in social situations out of nervousness. Or perhaps your family or circle of friends encourages you to overeat, and it's easier to go along with the group.*

Stop emotional eating tip 2: Find other ways to feed your feelings

If you don't know how to manage your emotions in a way that doesn't involve food, you won't be able to control your eating habits for very long. Diets so often fail because they offer logical nutritional advice, as if the only thing keeping you from eating right is knowledge. But that kind of advice only works if you have conscious control over your eating habits. It doesn't work when emotions hijack the process, demanding an immediate payoff with food.

In order to stop emotional eating, you have to find other ways to fulfill yourself emotionally. It's not enough to understand the cycle of emotional eating or even to understand your triggers, although that's a huge first step. You need alternatives to food that you can turn to for emotional fulfillment.

Alternatives to emotional eating

- **If you're depressed or lonely,** call someone who always makes you feel better, play with your dog or cat, or look at a favorite photo or cherished memento.
- **If you're anxious,** expend your nervous energy by dancing to your favorite song, squeezing a stress ball, or taking a brisk walk.
- **If you're exhausted,** treat yourself with a hot cup of tea, take a bath, light some scented candles, or wrap yourself in a warm blanket.
- **If you're bored,** read a good book, watch a comedy show, explore the outdoors, or turn to an activity you enjoy (woodworking, playing the guitar, shooting hoops, scrapbooking, etc.).

Learn to practice mindful eating

Mindful eating is a practice that develops your awareness of eating habits and allows you to pause between your triggers and your actions.

- *Awareness of your physical and emotional cues*
- *Awareness of your non-hunger triggers for eating*
- *Awareness on how you buy, prepare and eat your food*
- *Choosing foods that give you both enjoyment and nourishment*
- *Learning to meet your emotional needs in ways other than eating*

Mindful eating tip: Pause when cravings hit

Most emotional eaters feel powerless over their food cravings. When the urge to eat hits, it's all you can think about. You feel an almost unbearable tension that demands to be fed, right now! Because you've tried to resist in the past and failed, you believe that your willpower just isn't up to snuff. But the truth is that you have more power over your cravings than you think.

Take 5 before you give in to a craving

Emotional eating tends to be automatic and virtually mindless. Before you even realize what you're doing, you've reached for a tub of ice cream and polished off half of it. But if you can take a moment to pause and reflect when you're hit with a craving, you give yourself the opportunity to make a different decision.

Can you put off eating for five minutes, or just start with one minute. Don't tell yourself you can't give in to the craving; remember, the forbidden is extremely tempting. Just tell yourself to wait. While you're waiting, check in with yourself. How are you feeling? What's going on emotionally? Even if you end up eating, you'll have a better understanding of why you did it. This can help you set yourself up for a different response next time.

Learn to accept your feelings—even the bad ones

While it may seem that the core problem is that you're powerless over food, emotional eating actually stems from feeling powerless over your emotions. You don't feel capable of dealing with your feelings head on, so you avoid them with food.

Allowing yourself to feel uncomfortable emotions can be scary. You may fear that, like Pandora's box, once you open the door you won't be able to shut it. But the truth is that when we don't obsess over or suppress our emotions, even the most painful and difficult feelings subside relatively quickly and lose their power to control our attention. To do this you need to become mindful and learn how to stay connected to your moment-to-moment emotional experience. This can enable you to rein in stress and repair emotional problems that often trigger emotional eating.

8 steps to mindful eating

This ancient practice can transform the way you think about food and set the stage for a lifetime of healthy eating.

Like most of us, you've probably eaten something in the past few hours. And, like many of us, you may not be able to recall everything you ate, let alone the *sensation of eating it.* Because we're working, driving, reading, watching television, or fiddling with an electronic device, we're not fully aware of what we're eating.

By truly paying attention to the food you eat, you may indulge in foods like a cheeseburger and fries less often. In essence, mindful eating means being fully attentive to your food—as you buy, prepare, serve, and consume it. In the book *Savor: Mindful Eating, Mindful Life*, Dr. Lillian Cheung and her co-author, Buddhist spiritual leader Thich Nhat Hanh, suggest several practices that can help you get there, including those listed below.

1. **Begin with your shopping list.** Consider the health value of every item you add to your list and stick to it to avoid impulse buying when you're shopping. Fill most of your cart in the produce section and avoid the center aisles—which are heavy with processed foods—and the chips and candy at the check-out counter.
2. **Come to the table with an appetite—but not when ravenously hungry.** If you skip meals, you may be so eager to get anything in your stomach that your first priority is filling the void instead of enjoying your food.
3. **Start with a small portion.** It may be helpful to limit the size of your plate to nine inches or less.
4. **Appreciate your food.** Pause for a minute or two before you begin eating to contemplate everything and everyone it took to bring the meal to your table. Silently express your gratitude for the opportunity to enjoy delicious food and the companions you're enjoying it with.
5. **Bring all your senses to the meal.** When you're cooking, serving, and eating your food, be attentive to color, texture, aroma, and even the sounds different foods make as you prepare them. As you chew your food, try identifying all the ingredients, especially seasonings.
6. **Take small bites.** It's easier to taste food completely when your mouth isn't full. Put down your utensil between bites.

7. ***Chew thoroughly.*** *Chew well until you can taste the essence of the food. (You may have to chew each mouthful 20 to 40 times, depending on the food.) You may be surprised at all the flavors that are released.*
8. ***Eat slowly.*** *If you follow the advice above, you won't bolt your food down. Devote at least five minutes to mindful eating before you chat with your tablemates.*

CHAPTER 100

GETTING STARTED

How do you get your family to go from eating the standard American diet to a whole food, plant based diet? I think the best way is by small, baby steps. I started by replacing meat with grains. I used ¼ grain with ¾ meat, then ½ and ½, and then inverse to ¾ grain and ¼ meat, until the meat was totally gone. You can use any grain; just precook it, and add it to your meat as you cook it. Meat was the easiest thing for our family to give up, which is odd because we were eating so much of it for dinner in the past.

For cow's milk, find a substitute like almond milk, coconut milk, rice milk, soy milk or cashew milk. I make our cashew milk. It's so easy and delicious! I use it whenever I used cow's milk in the past. Check out my recipe section to see how easy it is to make.

Cheese has been hard for our family to give up, and some members of our family are still trying to let go. I learned to make a cashew cheese that most of us are okay with; we eat those or no cheese at all. Of course, there's that one adorable boy of mine who is here to make sure I understand what some of you might go through when changing the family diet. I love him! In *The China Study*, Dr. Campbell says you can turn cancer off when you keep your animal protein intake to 5% or less. My goal for my family has been 5% or less animal protein; but for me, it's 0%. Personally, I would rather have 0% chance of increasing my risk of disease. With all I've been through physically, it's not worth it for me to eat food that would cause me any more suffering down the road.

I'm not sure about your neighborhood, but everyone in sunny San Diego seems to have a pool and chickens! We missed out on the pool but we did have chickens. I used to think eggs were okay to eat as long as they were organic eggs. I have learned otherwise, so we don't eat eggs anymore. Instead we use chia seeds or flax seeds or Ener-G egg replacer when baking, and no one misses the eggs. I'm quite surprised that no one in the family even seemed to notice. We used to eat scrambled eggs a lot. Cool!

Changing the family diet is a process. Slow and steady worked best for me. We were having burritos for dinner, and I asked my 12-year-old if I could skip setting out the cheese and sour cream when we were first changing our diet. She said "Sure! Let's do this!" I shouted for joy. I could have forced this way of life on my kids, but I wanted it to happen by teaching them so that they would understand the reasoning and choose for themselves. I didn't want them to eat healthy food only when mom was watching.

Figure out what will work best for you and your family. For me, personally, I picked a date and started and never looked back; but I was informed and motivated. If I was a kid and this change was happening in my house, I know I'd prefer a slow shift as my taste buds and willingness adjusted. As time went on, my family ate less and less of the foods that are not whole food, plant based, and I'm so grateful for that.

Jane Birch, author of Discovering The Word Of Wisdom[239] really helped me get on track with a whole food, plant based diet. I am so grateful for her inspiration, kindness and willingness to share what she's learned. Here are her tips for making the transition easy.

Whole Food, Plant-Based (WFPB) Made Easy[240]

WFPB food preparation very naturally becomes easier the more you do it. Don't despair if it takes time at first. Make it an adventure/hobby, at least for a few weeks! It takes time for your taste buds to change and to find the foods you love and learn to make them just right. Once you have a few meals you love and know how to prepare, the bulk of the work is over. As you continue to make these same meals and experiment with new ones, you'll very quickly figure out ways to make food preparation VERY manageable.

People have a tendency to over-think and complicate WFPB cooking when they first start. Take it one week at a time. Don't start worrying now about Thanksgiving, the Church potluck or your summer family reunion. By keeping it simple and taking it one step at a time, you'll soon develop the skills you need for any situation.

Here are some top strategies for saving time:

- *Plan at least a week in advance so you can do all your shopping at once.*
- *Cook foods in large quantities so you have lots of leftovers. (As a single person, I can usually prepare 3–6 days' worth of food at one time. I keep some in the freezer.)*
- *Use some frozen vegetables and fruits and some canned goods like tomatoes and beans. These are already chopped and can save lots of time. The nutrient loss (if any) is minimal compared to the time saved.*
- *Find a few recipes or meals you like and repeat these over and over so you are not constantly trying new recipes. The average family needs only 6-8 recipes.*
- *Instead of relying on new recipes for variety, use the same recipes but change them up by swapping ingredients, like alternative vegetables, grains, or spices.*
- *Most recipes are forgiving. You don't need to run to the store to get "every" ingredient listed! Experiment with substitutions or just leave things out.*
- *Find some tricks to "saving" almost any meal if it does not turn out as good as you hoped. Some of my standbys include hot sauce (like Tabasco sauce), jalapeños (or other peppers), salsa, fruit, or even a little more salt.*
- *Use simple meal templates instead of recipes (see below).*

Using Simple Meal Templates

There are thousands of WFPB recipes you can find in fancy cookbooks or free on the Internet. Many of them are wonderful, but they sometimes require good cooking skills, lots of ingredients, and plenty of time. Whether you are a fantastic cook or just a novice, a great alternative is to use simple templates to prepare foods. Please remember: if you are just starting out, it may take a few weeks for your taste buds to adjust; don't get discouraged; keep moving forward in faith!

BASIC BREAKFAST TEMPLATE

1. Cook any whole grain (cracked or bulgar wheat; 5, 7, or 10-grain cereal; rolled, Scottish, or steel cut oats; brown rice; quinoa, etc.). Make a big batch to last many days.
2. For sweet cereals, add fruit (and a little sweetener if needed) along with a low-fat non-dairy milk (rice, soy, almond, etc.).
3. For a savory breakfast, add some veggies cooked in a little soy sauce or other favorite sauce.

BASIC LUNCH OR DINNER TEMPLATE

1. Choose a starch.
2. Add whatever vegetables you like.
3. Use sauces and/or spices for added flavor.
4. Have a piece of fruit for dessert.

More details on these basic templates:

1. Choose a starch. One of the keys to successfully switching to a WFPB diet is to eat enough whole starch foods. These foods are key to good health, weight control, and avoiding hunger. Make any one (or a combination) of these starches at least half your plate:

Whole grains: barley, oats, brown rice, quinoa, wheat berries (whole wheat kernels), buckwheat, rye, bulgur (a type of cracked wheat), triticale, corn, wild rice, millet. (Add 2-3 parts water to one part grain and cook until the water is mostly absorbed.)

Roots: white potatoes, sweet potatoes, celeriac (celery root), tapioca, Jerusalem artichoke, taro root, jicama, parsnips, rutabaga. (Steam or boil on the stove, bake in the oven, or cook in a microwave.)

Winter squashes: butternut, acorn, hubbard, banana, pumpkin, buttercup, turban squash. (Steam or boil on the stove, bake in the oven, or cook in a microwave.)

Legumes: Beans (adzuki, red kidney, black, mung, fava/broad, navy, garbanzo, pink, great northern, pinto, limas, white kidney/ cannellini); Lentils (brown, red, green); Peas (black-eyed, split yellow, split green, whole green). (You can buy these frozen or in cans or cook them yourself—cook in large quantities and freeze in small bags.)

2. Add vegetables. Add one or many more vegetables to your liking (for weight loss, add A LOT in volume!). There are so many to choose from. Vary them week-by-week for different flavors and nutrients if you like. Don't worry if you don't like most vegetables. Just start with what you like. Here are easy ways to cook them:

- Sauté without oil (use water, vegetable broth or any other non-oil liquid instead).
- Steam on the stove.
- Microwave (you can use any container, but I like using a silicone container with a lid).
- Roast in oven (instead of oil, try balsamic vinegar, oil-free sauce, or juice).
- Boil in water (you lose more nutrients this way, but you should be eating so many vegetables that the nutrients you lose won't make a difference health-wise).
- Eat raw.

How to sauté onions without oil:

1. Use a good non-stick pan (like Berndes or Swiss Diamond) or a high quality regular pan (and watch it more carefully). Let it get hot.

2. To a hot, dry pan, add chopped onion and allow it to start to brown. It may appear to stick a little but let it get brown and caramelize without adding any water (otherwise you will start poaching the onion instead of sautéing).
3. Once it starts to get brown, add a couple of tablespoons of non-oil liquid (e.g. water, juice, broth) but not too much (to avoid cooling the pan). The water added will bubble and steam.
4. Immediately mix the onions around the pan with a non-metal spatula, using the small amount of water just added to collect the brown, caramelized contents from the sides of the pan.
5. Add another couple of tablespoons of water to the pan and repeat the same process until the onions are brown and caramelized.

3. Use sauces and/or spices. The possibilities here are endless! Don't be afraid to try new things.

Spices. Experiment with different spices and spice mixes (like Mrs. Dash or Table Tasty Salt Substitute.)

Sauces. There are lots of WFPB recipes for sauces. There are also many sauces you can buy that fit the whole food, plant-based guidelines. Study the labels carefully to avoid animal foods and minimize sugar, salt, oil, and food additives. Here are sauces you can easily find:

- Salsas (there is a huge variety you can buy or you can easily make your own).
- Hot sauces (HUGE variety). I think Tabasco sauce spices up any dish.
- Mustard (many varieties).
- Vinegar (many varieties).
- Soy sauce, tamari, or Bragg's Amino Acids (get low-sodium varieties).
- Vegetable or fruit relishes.

This **Walnut Sauce recipe** is as easy and delicious as they get. Almost everyone I know loves it. I use it on rice, potatoes, and any cooked vegetables.

Walnut Sauce

Mix these ingredients in a food processor or blender:

1 cup walnut pieces
1 cup water
2–3 garlic cloves
2–4 tablespoons low sodium soy sauce or tamari sauce

4. Enjoy fruit for dessert. *Once you have stopped eating sugary desserts, the fruit will taste sweet and satisfying.*

Popular Food Templates

The following templates are well known to all of us. It is easy to be creative and find endless variety with little effort or just make it simple with 3–4 ingredients! Don't make it too complicated. Remember you can use frozen or canned veggies and beans and pre-cooked or frozen grains.

Note how each of these templates is a variation on the basic template: (1) starch; (2) vegetables; (3) sauces/spices.

Sandwiches or pitas. *Get good whole grain vegan bread or pita bread with little or no added oil. Add your favorite veggies, like cucumber, tomatoes, lettuce, mushrooms, and sprouts. Mustard or low-fat hummus works great as a spread.*

Burritos, tortillas, and tacos. *Find whole wheat, brown rice, whole spelt, or corn tortillas. Fill with rice and/or beans or sweet potatoes and veggies. Top with shredded lettuce, tomatoes, red onion, black olives, etc. Use vegan taco seasoning or other Mexican spices if desired. Enjoy with salsa.*

Enchiladas. *Layer corn tortillas with beans, brown rice, enchilada sauce (homemade or store bought) and vegetables like onions, bell peppers, carrots, and zucchini.*

Rice and/or bean bowl. *This is an easy favorite for many people. You can season the beans with cumin or other spices. Add your favorite vegetables. Flavor them with soy sauce, salsa, enchilada sauce or another favorite sauce and top with green onions, cilantro, etc.*

Mexican gumbo. Mix together a can of kidney, pinto, and/or black beans (juice and all); a cup of corn (or not); and a can of fire roasted diced tomatoes. Heat and add hot sauce.

Soup. A good vegetable and/or bean or lentil soup can be very filling. This is great for weight-loss because of the amount of water.

Pasta. Use whole-grain pasta as much as possible. Make sure there are no eggs. Make or purchase low-fat vegan pasta sauce (like marinara) and add lots of cooked veggies.

Pizza. Find (or purchase) a low-fat whole grain crust. Top with pizza sauce, pineapple, and vegetables.

Stir-fry. Stir-fry veggies you love, like peppers, carrots, and onions. Try some Asian favorites: water chestnuts, garlic, bok choy, bean sprouts, cabbage, or tofu. Flavor with soy sauce or other Asian sauces (I love adding a little Mae Ploy sweet chili sauce or any garlic chili sauce). Serve with brown rice or whole grain noodles.

Baked potatoes or potato bar. There is a huge variety of potatoes and lots of ways to cook them: bake, boil, steam, pressure cook or even microwave. Top with tomatoes, beans, corn and/or any type of raw or cooked vegetable: green onions, mushrooms, sprouts, jalapeños, etc. There are many possible vegan toppings: salsa or pico de gallo, barbecue sauce, soup, chili, sauerkraut, kimchi, or favorite condiments.

Mashed potatoes. Add non-dairy milk or veggie broth as you mash them. You can also mix in garlic, nutritional yeast, and/or seasonings.

Baked parcels. Cook any combination of vegetables/beans/rice you like, wrapped in parchment paper. Season with spices, herbs, Italian sauce, chili peppers, soy sauce, etc. Bake about 45 min. at 360°.

Salad or salad bar. Choose your favorite veggies (adding fruit also works well). Include a starch: corn, beans, whole wheat bread or potatoes. If you are used to traditional fat-filled dressings, it may take some time to get used to non-oil dressings. Don't worry—your tastes will change! Here is a simple no-oil salad dressing I make that has worked very well for me:

3-2-1 Salad Dressing

Mix these ingredients:
3 tablespoons balsamic vinegar
2 tablespoons mustard of choice (I use Dijon)
1 tablespoon maple syrup

Snacks

Eating large meals will help cut down on the need to snack, but it is also good to have some healthy snacks around. Here are a few I like (note that most of these are more calorie dense, so keep that in mind if you want to lose weight quickly):

Fruit. This is the best! I especially love frozen grapes, YUM!

Microwaved popcorn. Put no more than ¼ cup of popcorn kernels into a small brown lunch bag; fold the top well, microwave until the popping slows way down. I like to spray some soy sauce on it for flavor. I sometimes also add some spices or nutritional yeast. This works well, but I've burned the popcorn enough times that I now use a microwavable popcorn popper. You can also use a hot air popcorn maker.

Potato slices. Microwave 5 minutes each side, or 20–25 minutes in the oven at 425°. Dip in no-oil hummus, salsa, or ketchup.

Corn tortillas. Cut into fourths, bake on a cookie sheet at 425° for ten minutes. Dip in salsa or a bean dip.

Raw veggies. Dip in a no-oil hummus.

Cold cereal. Choose a whole grain cereal with low sugar/fat.

Smoothies. Try making them green with lots of green leafy vegetables. Add crushed ice and a little fruit for sweetness. Experiment with non-dairy milks.

Here are some great examples from Lindsay Nixon's *The Happy Herbivore Guide to Plant-based Living*.[241]

Lindsay's template:

- *Grain/Potato + Bean/Tofu + Greens/Veg + Sauce*
  - *Brown Rice + Kale + Black Beans + Pineapple or Peach Salsa*
  - *Quinoa + Baby Spinach + White Beans + Strawberries + Balsamic Dressing*
  - *Pasta + Broccoli + Chickpeas + Marinara Sauce*
  - *Tortilla + Spinach + Tomato + Hummus*
  - *Quinoa + Chickpeas + Bell Pepper + Italian dressing*
  - *Sweet Potato + Black Beans + Corn + Enchilada Sauce*
  - *Potato + Kale + Chickpeas + Gravy*
  - *Brown Rice + Black Eyed Peas + Corn + BBQ Sauce*
  - *Brown Rice + Frozen Mixed Veg + Tofu or Edamame + Soy Sauce*
  - *Quinoa + Tempeh + Pineapple + Teriyaki Sauce*

Lindsay suggests, "You can expand on any of these by adding sliced green onions or diced red onion, or another vegetable (cherry tomatoes pretty much go with anything) . . . If you can open a can, you can make these meals— and you can make them in the time it takes you to open the can. You can find precooked grains (like quinoa or brown rice) on the shelf or freezer of any store and they take a minute or two to heat up. Canned beans just need a rinse. The vegetables might need a moment in the microwave or steamer and the same for the sauces."

Meals and Meals Plans You Can Purchase

- *PlantPure Jumpstart*[242] *(continental United States)*
- *Happy Herbivore: 7-day Meal Plans*[243] *(anywhere)*

What I Eat

I am not a cook. I really mean that. You cannot be a worse cook than I am. When I first started this diet, I struggled so much that I finally got on the McDougall Discussion Board to plead for help. Others with experience responded with lots of great recipes and other ideas for succeeding. You can still read the posts here: "Help! I'm NOT enjoying my new food.[244]"

It took me awhile, but after a few weeks, my taste buds changed, and I figured out what I liked. Since then, I've LOVED the food! If I can do this, ANYONE (over the age of 12) can do this. There are many wonderful foods you can eat on this diet. My way is extremely simple, and it works for me. Here is what I normally eat:

Breakfast: *a whole grain, hot cereal (cracked or bulgur wheat; 5, 7, or 10-grain cereal; rolled, Scottish, or steel cut oats; brown rice; quinoa, etc.). My favorite is steel cut oats. I top it with chopped fresh fruit and frozen banana for sweetening and use non-dairy milk. I am also adding a tablespoon of ground flax seed. This is all so delicious that before I go to bed each night, I'm already looking forward to breakfast!*

You can cook whole grain cereals in the microwave, a slow cooker, pressure cooker, or rice cooker. On stovetop: Bring 2–3 parts water to boil, add 1-part grain, and turn down heat to low as you stir; then cover and cook for 10-30 minutes (depending on how chewy you like your cereal) without opening the lid (make sure you turn down the heat low enough that it won't boil over). With a very large pan, you can make enough cereal to last you quite a few days, then just reheat in the microwave each day. I make one big batch (6 cups of dry oats) a week and then microwave a HUGE serving every morning in a silicone container.

Lunch and Dinner: *My meals usually have three parts:*

A starch. *I make a starch item the center of each meal. My favorite is different varieties of brown rice. I cook a large batch in a top-of-the-line Asian rice cooker. The cooker does make a difference. Get an Asian brand, like the Korean Cuckoo.*

Beans. *I use a variety over time. Beans are inexpensive; buy low-sodium beans in cans (drain and rinse before using). They are even cheaper if you cook them yourself in a pressure cooker or slow cooker. I cook a big batch in a pressure cooker and then freeze them in small bags. I often add dry (or soaked) beans to the dry rice before cooking the rice.*

Veggies. These also vary widely, and I often have two to four kinds on my plate, though one is enough. I typically steam or sauté them, but they can also be boiled, roasted, or microwaved. You can experiment with adding spices, but I'm not very good at that. I do like to sauté some garlic and onion in a little water or vegetable broth; then after it is cooked, I add the vegetable and continue to cook until done, maybe adding some low-sodium tamari (a Japanese soy sauce) and chili garlic sauce. Adding tomatoes also works for me since I like juicy foods.

Note: I use no sodium or very low sodium ingredients and add no salt while cooking, but then I sometimes add salt once the food is on my plate. I often use some "walnut sauce" on the veggies and/or beans and rice (see recipe above). I love to add fruit to my meals or eat afterward as dessert. I also frequently have a very large salad for a meal (greens, a few veggies, garbanzo beans, fruit, etc.) with the 3-2-1 dressing (see above). I'm addicted to arugula! I also eat other foods, but the above is my mainstay.

Treats. I often eat healthy snacks that are not calorie dense, but I occasionally eat a sparing amount of more calorie dense foods for a treat (e.g. dried fruit, whole grain cold cereal, fruit smoothies, nuts, WFPB cookies, avocado). I know people on a SAD diet who are trying to include more of these types of foods into their diet because they are so much healthier than SAD. So, for some people, these are the healthiest foods they eat, whereas for me, they are the richest foods I eat.

CHAPTER 101

RECIPES AND COOKING TIPS

THE KEY TO cooking is keeping it simple. You really don't even need recipes. Grains, beans, legumes, potatoes, corn, sweet potatoes, fruits and veggies are all you need. If you want to make things a bit fancier or your family is hoping that you will, check out some of my recipes in the following section.

On trick I use at the store is that I read the ingredients on something that looks yummy, or the ingredients of something my family ate in the past, and now I make my own healthier version. A perfect example is my cashew ranch dressing. I used soaked cashews and water for the base and then added the healthy ingredients that were on the back of the ranch dressing bottle such as parsley, mustard, and vinegar. It turned out great! You can find that recipe in the following recipe section too. Cooking should be fun and creative. If recipes hold you back, skip them and create your own.

It's great to use heavy duty stainless steel pots so you can use water or vegetable broth to sauté your food and avoid all that excess fat from oils which damages your cells, leading to lots of health trouble. I also love my ceramic skillet, which I use for pancakes.

I learned to mill my own flour from Chef Brad on the BYU-TV show "Fusion Grain Cooking." Chef Brad makes what he calls "WonderFlour[245]" by milling spelt, barley and brown rice. I really enjoy this combination and use this homemade flour for all my cooking and baking. I had a hand mill that really made me feel like a pioneer, but it would literally take our family a week to mill enough grain for one loaf of bread. An electric grain mill is relatively inexpensive, especially if you are buying organic flours. I make a large batch by milling three to four cups of each grain all at once and it takes about five minutes to turn into fresh, homemade whole grain flour. After that, I have enough flour for all my cooking and baking for two weeks or more. I put the flour in a gallon zip lock bag in the freezer and pull it out for use as I need it during the week. I don't make everything from scratch, but almost everything. I do buy spelt bread, as our family goes through it faster than I can make it!

Make sure you buy aluminum free baking powder. Why eat aluminum when you can avoid it!

Slice parchment paper into strips and lay them across the muffin tins for non-stick muffin baking. They are easier to peel than paper muffin cups.

Always eat organic if you can. Why eat chemicals and pesticides if you can avoid it? Remember that a non-organic vegetable is still much healthier for you than an animal product.

Use a salt that has minerals in it, like sea salt or pink Himalayan salt, not refined table salt.

When you buy green onions, use them and save the unused base of the stalks and put them in water to re-grow in your kitchen window or replant in your garden. They seem to just keep producing! My water-planted window green onions don't like the summer window heat and the water starts to stink. Once that happens, I replant them outside.

I have a few favorite spices that I seem to use on everything. Because each food has its own unique flavor, everything I make does not taste the same! My favorite spices are onion and garlic granules, minced garlic, and pink Himalayan salt. Cook anything in onion and garlic and it taste pretty darn good. Sprinkle a bit of salt on top when you are done cooking and you've got something delicious, even if it's just some grilled veggies— which are actually one of my favorites!

I also use a ton of green onions. I also use lots of cilantro and parsley as well. So fresh, healthy, flavorful and beautiful.

I love chia seeds and put them in almost everything I bake and any breakfast I make. Delicious, crunchy and awesome brain power food!

BREAKFAST

Favorite Breakfast Pancakes
4 cups of your favorite whole grain flour or a mix of flours. I mill barley, spelt and brown rice. I learned that from Chef Brad. He calls this mix WonderFlour.[246] I use it for all my baking.
½ cup chia seeds
¼ cup 100% pure maple syrup
1 tbsp. cinnamon
3 tbsp. baking powder
Egg replacer for 4 eggs
4 cups filtered water
Stir all ingredients and throw on a hot ceramic griddle. Serve with berries and applesauce and more maple syrup if you like it even sweeter.

Quinoa Lemon Delight
4 cups cooked quinoa chilled (any color or multicolor quinoa is fine)
2 cups organic unfiltered apple juice
1 tsp. cinnamon
1 tsp. vanilla
½ cup slivered almonds
1 whole organic lemon plus the zest (if you like zest) (minus the seeds)
1 cup Craisins™ or raisins
Stir and enjoy!

French Toast
8 slices of your favorite whole grain bread
Ener-G egg replacer for the equivalent of 2 eggs
2 cups nondairy milk like nut milk, soy milk or rice milk

1 tsp. cinnamon
½ tsp. vanilla
3 tbsp. 100% pure maple syrup (Don't use agave as it's extra sticky and burns)

Get out your favorite non-stick pan; ceramic is the best I've found so far because the coating on the pan is not toxic. Turn the heat to medium, and let the pan warm up to hot while you mix up the French toast ingredients. In a bowl, add the water and egg replacer as directed on the box for the equivalent of two eggs. Then add the non-dairy milk of your choice. Our favorite is vanilla cashew milk (homemade is best, and oh so easy). Then add the vanilla, cinnamon, maple syrup and mix. Dip the bread into the mix soaking both sides of the bread and put it on the hot pan. With a good metal spatula and a little loving care, flip the toast once it's browned on one side and cook until it's no longer soggy. Serve with fruit and a bit more maple syrup to taste.

Oatmeal (or any hot grain cereal) Topped with Fruit
Most grains are cooked with 1 cup of grains in 2 cups of water. After cooking, top with fresh fruit, cinnamon, nut milk and 100% pure maple syrup.

Cold Cereal
Look for oil free, whole grain organic cereals. The less ingredients the better. Or try your hand at making your own!

Pecan Banana Muffins
What can you do with all those overripe bananas sitting on your counter? Try this!

6 overripe bananas
4 cups of your favorite whole grain flour

2 tbsp. aluminum free baking powder
1 tsp. vanilla
3 tbsp. chia seeds
½ cup 100% pure maple syrup
1 cup organic apple sauce
Ener-G egg replacer to the equivalent of 4 eggs
1 cup water
1 cup chopped pecans or your favorite nut

Pre-heat your oven to 350 degrees. With a fork, squish the ripe bananas in your mixing bowl. Next add all other ingredients and mix. Scoop the mix into muffin papers in a muffin tin or slice parchment paper into strips and lay them across the muffin tins to keep the muffins from sticking. Bake for 25-30 minutes until golden brown. Serve hot!

LUNCH

Veggie Sandwiches
We love these sandwiches and my daughters take them for school lunch all the time! They are also one of our favorite quick meals after church on Sundays when we all come home hungry.

2 slices of oil free whole grain bread
Light layer of avocado, or cashew cheese on one slice of bread
Light or heavy layer of mustard on the other slice
One extra-large, thick sliced tomato
Thin layer of cucumber
1 handful of alfalfa sprouts
One large lettuce leaf
*Optional—pickle slices and peppers of any type.

Tostadas, Soft Tacos or Mexican Bowl
I love Mexican food! I'm pretty sure there is nothing better. It's so easy to make as well. Since I've given you a few types of dishes here, there will be some options. The base and fixings are the same for each. Just the tortillas are different.

Base:
Whole pinto or black beans or fat free refried pinto beans.
Brown rice
Lettuce
Tomato
Salsa
*Optional—cilantro, grilled fajita-type mix of peppers and onions or spicy carrots, onion and jalapenos, avocado or guacamole, and cashew cheese for extra rich flavor.

For the tortilla, I use non-GMO organic corn tortillas that are just corn and water. You can warm them for a soft taco, bake them on a cookie sheet on high broil for about 3 minutes then flip and cook another 3 minutes until they are crispy. You know you waited too long to check on them when the fire alarm rings. Our family joke is that the fire alarm is the dinner bell. Ha, ha. Most flour tortillas have fat in them, lard or some type of oil. Best to avoid those if you can.

Beans are cheap to make yourself but you've got to plan ahead a bit. Soak your beans overnight and then cook them for about 90 minutes on the stovetop, or 30 minutes in a pressure cooker. Drain, and turn them to refried beans by adding some water and blending with an immersion blender. You could also mash your beans by putting your beans and water in a high powered blender or food processor. If you are in a rush, grab a can of fat free organic refried beans.

Rice and Asian Veggies with Spicy Sauce + Tofu Fry
We love stir fry! I especially love the spicy sauce. This recipe is quick and easy.

2 cups white rice
2 bags frozen stir fry veggies
4 tbsp. water
Any additional veggies that you want; mushrooms, baby corn, bamboo shoots, water chestnuts
4 tbsp. tamari sauce or soy sauce

We eat this recipe a lot as it only takes about 15 minutes to make. You can use brown rice, and you'll double your cooking time but add nutrition, so I'll leave that up to you. Cook the rice as directed on the package. Add your frozen veggies to a large stainless steel skillet. Turn the heat to medium and immediately add the water so you don't burn your veggies. Add any non-frozen additional veggies after your frozen veggies have thawed a bit. Add the tamari sauce (now start your spicy sauce while the veggies warm up) and simmer until steaming hot. Serve over a bed of rice and top with spicy sauce.

Tofu Dry Fry
Recently we tried a tofu dry fry and love it. Give it a try and add a new flavor and texture to your meals!
1 package 20oz. firm tofu
½ cup rice vinegar
¼ cup soy sauce
3 tbps. 100% pure maple syrup

Drain and cube the firm tofu and marinate in a mixture of rice vinegar, soy sauce and 100% pure maple syrup. Put cubed tofu and marinade in a zip lock bag on the counter to marinate for 20-30 minutes.

Pour tofu and marinade in a stainless pan and cook until liquids are absorbed. If you have less time, drain marinade before the dry fry. Brown all sides of the tofu and enjoy on your stir-fry.

Spicy Sauce
1 box vegetable broth
3 tbsp. corn starch
4 tbsp. hot Asian garlic and red pepper sauce

The spicy sauce is so simple! In another smaller stainless steel sauce pan, add a box of vegetable broth and the flour to thicken the sauce. It won't get thick immediately so don't keep adding flour and turn your sauce solid. Ha! Turn the heat to medium and continue stirring frequently. Make sure to add the corn starch to the sauce before it gets hot or it will stay clumpy. If you need to add cornstarch late I the game, mix it with cold water first to avoid the clumps. Add the garlic red pepper sauce any time before it comes to a boil. Once it boils reduce heat and simmer for one minute. Enjoy!

Farro Jicama Salad
4 cups cooked farro (grain)
1 cup chopped jicama
1 chopped fresh jalapeño
1 cup chopped tomatoes
1 cup chopped bell peppers (choose your color or use a mix)
½ cup chopped parsley
Juice from one lemon
¼ cup fig balsamic vinegar

Cook farro which is a wheat grain as directed on the package and cool. Chop your favorite veggies like jicama, jalapeño, tomatoes, and bell peppers. Chop some parsley too. Serve in a buffet line. Grab a plate of farro and choose your toppings. Top with fresh squeezed lemon juice and fig balsamic vinegar. Sweet, sour, spicy, crispy, light, hearty, healthy, pretty, fast and so tasty! Enjoy!

Cilantro and Wild Rice Salad

Here is a wonderful, fast, easy, delicious, nutritious, beautiful and hardy rice salad. Serve with pasta, grilled vegetables or potatoes. Make sure to bring this salad to your next gathering. It's so pretty!

3 cups cooked brown rice
1 cup cooked wild rice
1 can rinsed black beans
1 cup thawed frozen peas
1 cup thawed frozen corn
½ cup green onions
½ cup chopped fresh cilantro
¼ tsp pink Himalayan salt
1 dash of pepper

Really, you can eat this salad warm or cold. I've done it both ways. If you are cooking your rice at the time you make the salad, it's easier to eat it warm so you don't have to cool the rice. Grab a bowl, add all ingredients on the list, stir and eat. Easy peasy!

SIDES, SAUCES, AND MORE

Tortilla Chips

Organic, non-GMO corn tortillas
Pink Himalayan salt

Get some organic non-GMO corn tortillas. Turn the oven to high broil. Cut the tortillas like a pizza. Lay them on a cookie tray with a light sprinkle of salt. Put them in the oven for about 5 minutes checking frequently that they are not burning. Pull them out and flip them over and then put them back in the oven for about another 4 minutes still checking frequently to keep them from burning. They are most crispy when they are well toasted. If you pull them out too soon they are a bit chewy and no one likes chewy chips! Serve with your favorite salsa. I like to make a few cookie sheets full of chips before I announce there are chips in the kitchen as the kids eat them faster than I can make them and then we are all left staring at the oven.

Salsa
In a food processor, add some ripe tomatoes, onions (white or green,) cilantro, garlic and jalapeño slices if you like it hot. Puree and serve. Delicious! You can also add some lemon or lime, salt, and canned tomatoes for a sweeter taste. If you like a greener salsa, add more cilantro.

Quick and Easy Veggie Pasta Sauce
The other night I was making a pasta dish and wanted to make up a new sauce. It turned out great and was so fun that I did it again the following night and loved that one too. Here are my two new favorite pasta sauces if we are not using an oil free marinara.

Cauliflower Pesto Sauce
½ cup veggie broth
1 tsp. minced garlic
1 whole cauliflower
¼ cup fresh chopped basil
1 tsp. pink Himalayan salt
½ cup water

In a large stainless steel saucepan on medium heat, add the vegetable broth and minced garlic. While that simmers wash and chop the cauliflower and add to the saucepan. Next go to your garden and grab and large handful of basil leave. If you are a basil lover grab more than one handful. Wash and chop the basil and add to the saucepan along with the salt. Simmer on low until cauliflower is soft. Pour whole hot mixture into a blender and add one cup of warm water. Blend until smooth and pour over your favorite pasta.

Vegan Cheesy Zucchini Sauce
½ cup veggie broth
1 tsp. minced garlic
2 zucchinis, about 8 inches long
1 cup nutritional yeast
1 tsp. pink Himalayan salt
½ cup water

In a large stainless steel saucepan on medium heat, add the vegetable broth and minced garlic. While that simmers wash and chop the zucchini and add to the saucepan. Simmer on low until zucchini is soft. Pour whole hot mixture into a blender and nutritional yeast (for the cheesy flavor) and warm water. Blend until smooth and pour over your favorite pasta.

Cheesy Cauliflower Sauce
½ cup veggie broth
1 tsp. minced garlic
1 whole cauliflower
2 yellow squash, about 8 inches long
1 cups nutritional yeast
1 tsp. pink Himalayan salt
½ cup water

In a large stainless steel saucepan on medium heat, add the vegetable broth and minced garlic. While that simmers wash and chop the cauliflower and yellow squash and add to the saucepan. Simmer on medium heat until the veggies are soft. Pour hot veggie mixture into a blender and nutritional yeast (for the cheesy flavor). Add the salt and veggie water from the cooked veggie pan. If your blender is having a hard time mixing, add a bit more water but not too much because it's so yummy thick and creamy! Blend until smooth and pour over your favorite pasta. This is a favorite!!!

Cashew Ranch Dressing
In an attempt to get my family off all animal products and oils, ranch dressing has been a battle. Ranch dressing is so good for dipping veggies! I finally came up with a recipe that the whole family loves. I also served it at a realtor's open house the other day with a veggie tray, and I was told I should bottle it and sell it. Yay, they like it! It's still high fat and not recommended if you are trying to slim down or have heart issues, but if you are going to dip your veggies in ranch anyway, and don't have a cashew allergy, try this recipe instead!

2 cups soaked cashew nuts
2-3 cups water, depending on how thick you like it
1 tsp. dried parsley
2 tbsp. white vinegar
1 tbsp. yellow mustard
½ tsp. pink salt

Wash the cashews, then soak them for at least 4 hours but overnight is even better. Soak in cool filtered water. Cashews almost double in size, so use enough water. After soaking, drain and rinse the nuts and put them into a food processor with water. The dressing tends to thicken even more once you make it so keep that in mind. Blend until smooth, scraping down the sides of the food processor any nut pieces that are not mixing in. Add: dried parsley (this ingredient gives it the traditional specked ranch look,) white vinegar, yellow mustard, and pink salt. Process until very smooth, adding any additional water that might be needed. Poor into a salad dressing type bottle or mason jar with a lid and refrigerate or grab some veggies and enjoy!

Sunflower & Green Onion Oil-Free Hummus
We all love to dip veggies! But what dip is healthy? That is the question. Hummus is a great option, but let's make it without oil, which is a processed food, not a health food. Try my new favorite hummus creation.

1 can garbanzo beans
½ tsp. onion granules
½ tsp. garlic granules
½ tsp. pink Himalayan salt
4 tbsp. nutritional yeast
¾ cup water
1 tbsp. sunflower seeds
1 tbsp. diced green onions

In a food processor with a chopping blade, add rinsed garbanzo beans, onion granules, garlic granules, pink Himalayan salt, nutritional yeast, water and blend for 1 minute. Scoop hummus into a decorative plate or bowl, then sprinkle with sunflower seeds and diced green onions. Add more or less sunflower seeds and diced green onion to taste and beauty. Serve with your favorite veggies and enjoy!

Nut Milk for All Your Recipes
4-5 cups filtered water
1 cup raw washed nuts
optional—½ tsp. of vanilla

Get out your high powered blender and add the water (use 4-5 cups depending on how thick you like your milk,) nuts and optional vanilla and blend on a smoothie type setting. Make sure the blender lid is on tight—I learned that one the hard way! Adding vanilla is delicious if it's milk for baking or breakfast. Skip the vanilla if it's a dinner recipe. We accidentally used the vanilla milk in mashed potatoes twice now! Oops! Pour the milk through cheesecloth and squeeze all the milk out and discard of the pulp, or compost or use in another recipe like a nut cheese. Enjoy immediately or refrigerate. Cheap (buy your nuts on sale,) simple and no preservatives or oils like the store sells. So tasty too!

Cashew Cheese
Giving up cheese was really hard on our family. I'd be lying if I said all six of us are cheese free. In an attempt to soften the blow of giving up a Harkleroad all-time favorite food, I've found a cashew cheese recipe that my family loves. We use this cheese on toast, garlic bread, burritos, enchiladas, veggie sandwiches, etc. Anything we used to put cheese on, we can replace with this cheese. Ok, not on soup, but there are ways to make that too.

2 cups raw cashews
1 cup water
1 probiotic capsule
1 cheese cloth
1 tsp. garlic powder
1 tsp. onion powder
½ tsp. pink salt (to taste)
4 tbsp.. nutritional yeast

This recipe takes several days to make depending on how hard you like your cheese so plan ahead. Don't let the timing scare you. It's not hard to make, we just need time for the probiotics to do their job and the cheese to harden if you don't want to use it like a spread.

Wash 2 cups of cashews, then soak them for at least 4 hours, but overnight is even better. If you let the nuts soak for days they will turn slimy. Yep, learned that one the hard way too. Soak in cool filtered water. Cashews almost double in size so use enough water. After soaking, drain and rinse and put the nuts into a food processor with one cup of water. Empty one probiotic capsule into the mix. Blend until very smooth, scraping down the sides of the food processor as needed to gather any runaway nut pieces! Get a bowl and set a strainer inside. Lay the cheese cloth into the strainer and pour the cheese mixture into the cheese cloth. Gather the corners of the cheese cloth and lift until you have a hanging ball of very, very soft cheese. Give it a light squeeze, getting a small amount of excess cashew milk from the mixture. Don't squeeze all the liquid out, just the excess with an easy squeeze. Set the cheese ball, while still wrapped in the cheese cloth, in the strainer. Set something heavy on top of the cheese like a can of food on top of a small bowl or plate. This will slowly squeeze the cheese. Make sure you keep it in the strainer with a bowl underneath. Cover the whole thing with a towel and leave on the counter for 24 hours while the probiotics do their thing. The following day, put the cheese back in the food processor and add the garlic powder, onion powder, pink salt and nutritional yeast. Blend again in the food processor until seasonings are mixed with the cheese. You can now eat the cheese as is with this cream cheese like consistency. Or you can wrap the cheese back in the cheese cloth and set on the counter on a plate or bowl to harden for 1-3 days. After 3 days, you can slice it but it's still a softer cheese. Our family likes this cheese in spreadable form. This recipe seems complex at first but now we make it by memory with ease.

Easy Salad Dressing
2 cups veggie broth and seasoning
3 tbsp. balsamic vinegar
2 tbsp. fresh ground flax seeds
*optional-1-2 tbsp. 100% pure organic maple syrup.

After sautéing any veggies and seasonings in a stainless steel pot, take out and cool the leftover juices and use them for a salad dressing base.

You could use leftover liquids from soups too, if you added too much liquid to your soup. Then add ground flax seeds to thicken the mixture, balsamic vinegar to give it a kick and if you like it sweet, a bit of maple syrup. Since your veggie stir fries, seasonings and soups are always different, your salad dressing will always be unique. Viola!

DINNER

15 Minute Mexican
4 cups quinoa
6 cups filtered water
2 tbsp. minced garlic
2 bunches of green onions
Fresh chopped jalapenos, if you like it hot
1 finely chopped zucchini
1 finely chopped yellow squash
1 can of organic low sodium pinto beans
1 can of organic low sodium white beans
1 can of organic low sodium kidney beans
1 can of organic low sodium black beans
2 cups of your favorite salsa

I'm not sure if your husband is like mine, but I never know when he will be home for dinner. Most days he's home late and I'm able to make dinner before he shows up, but once in a while he walks in early, so what can I make really fast that is yummy? Introducing my 15 Minute Mexican dish. Just a side note, my husband is happy to make his own food but I really like to do the cooking.

First, put some quinoa and water in a stainless steel sauté pan per cooking instruction on the package. In a large stainless steel skillet add a few tbsp. of water for sautéing the green onions, garlic, jalapenos, zucchini and squash. Once the veggies are cooked and tender add the canned beans. Make sure to rinse them with water first or they will turn your quinoa gray and it's just not as pretty. Top with your favorite salsa and then serve over your freshly made quinoa or serve inside some hot whole grain oil free tortillas. Ole!

Veggie Red Potato Soup and Bread
1 box low sodium organic vegetable broth
8 cups filtered water
1 yellow onion
6 celery stalks (this means 6 individual pieces of celery, not the whole head)
10 diced red potatoes
1 can of fire roast tomatoes
2 bay leaves
1 tbsp. pink Himalayan salt
1-2 diced yellow squash
1-2 diced zucchinis
3-4 cups cooked rice or grain of choice

I love soups and breads! I just can't get enough, especially in the winter. Soups are so easy to make and near impossible to mess up.

Start with a box of low sodium organic vegetable broth and water and then start chopping and adding the veggies and potatoes and all ingredients as the liquid heats up. Bring to a boil for about 15 minutes or until the veggies and potatoes are tender. Add your favorite leftover rice or cooked grains when the soup is done cooking. Best if served with homemade bread hot out of the oven. You could even drizzle the bread with honey. For a cheesy taste, sprinkle your soup with nutritional yeast. Yum!

Mashed Potatoes and Gravy
When it comes to comfort food, is there anything better than mashed potatoes and gravy? So satisfying and delicious and cheap and easy to make!

JENNY HARKLEROAD

Mashed Potatoes:
5 lb. bag organic potatoes (potatoes are on the dirty dozen list, which mean they are heavily sprayed with chemicals; so buy organic if you can, or grow your own!)
1 tbsp. pink Himalayan salt
3-4 cups of your favorite nondairy milk (Make sure you don't buy or make the milk vanilla flavor for your mashed potatoes!)

Gravy:
1 box of no oil, low sodium organic vegetable broth.
1 tsp. pink Himalayan salt
*optional-¼ tsp. pepper
½ tsp. parsley
½ tsp. garlic powder
½ tsp. onion powder
* add any of your favorite additional spices if you like your gravy herby
2 tbsp. cornstarch

Peel and dice your potatoes and throw them in a pot of boiling water uncovered for 30 minutes. Drain the potatoes and put them back in the pot. Add the salt, non-dairy milk and mix with a hand held mixer until smooth and creamy.

While the potatoes are cooking, get a medium sized stainless steel sauce pan and add all the gravy ingredients and mix before turning on the heat. The gravy will thicken as you cook it. Bring to a boil and then simmer for 1 minute stirring frequently.

Our family loves eating green peas and a side salad with our potatoes. Serve hot and enjoy!

Veggie Pizza
4 cups of your favorite whole grain flour or flour blend
3 cups warm water
½ cup chia seeds
1 packets of yeast

1 tbsp. baking soda
*optional-cashew cheese
1 jar oil free pasta sauce
4 cups of your favorite diced or sliced veggies pre-cooked
2 tsp. corn meal

Crust: Mix your favorite whole grain flour, warm water, chia seeds, yeast and baking soda. Cover the freshly made dough with a clean, warm and moist kitchen towel and let rise for one hour unless you are lucky enough to have a bread mixer and then you can run it for 6 minutes and you are ready to go!

Get a deep cookie sheet and sprinkle corn meal on the bottom to keep the crust from sticking, spread the crust around the pan with your hand. Get your hands very wet and flatten the dough with your hands. Each time the dough starts to stick to you, get your hands wet again until the dough is spread over your cookie sheet.

With a 425 degree preheated oven, bake the crust for 12 minutes or until golden brown. Remove from the oven and top your crust with the optional cashew cheese. Then top with an oil free, sugar free, low sodium marinara sauce.

In a stainless steel pan put all the chopped veggies you want on your pizza with some garlic and water for stir frying the veggies. If you put your veggies on the pizza uncooked and you like a ton of veggies like me, especially tomatoes, you will have some very soggy pizza! Drain the veggies (save veggie juice for future veggie sautéing or for your next salad dressing.) Top your pizza with your veggie mix.

Stick the pizza back in the oven for 10 more minutes at 425 degrees. Let cool for 5-10 minutes, Cut and serve. Yummy!

Delicious 3 Bean Chili
¼ cup minced garlic
3x 14oz cans of fire roasted tomatoes (2 processed in the recipe and one direct from the can later)
1 yellow onion

JENNY HARKLEROAD

1 bag of dry pinto beans soaked overnight
1 bag of dry white beans soaked overnight
1 bag of dry black beans soaked overnight
8 cups filtered water
1 small jar hot salsa
¼ cup taco seasoning
3 tbsp. chili powder
3 bunches of green onions

This makes a very large pot of chili, so cut the recipe if you are not feeding a large crowd or don't want to store the extras in the freezer.

In a Blendtec or other high powered blender add minced garlic, fire roasted diced tomatoes and one yellow onion. Blend until liquefied.

Soak the beans overnight in a pot of water. The beans will greatly increase in size, so make sure you use a big pot and lots of water. If you soak the beans they won't give you gas. Soak one bag of dry black beans, one bag of white beans and one bag of pinto beans.

Pour the soaked beans in a large pot and turn heat to medium high. Add contents of the blender plus filtered water. Add one small jar of hot salsa, taco seasoning and chili powder. Once the chili comes to a boil put on low and simmer for 2 hours stirring every 30 minutes. After 2 hours, add one can of fire roasted tomatoes not processed in the blender and chopped green onion. Simmer for 2 more hours stirring every 30 minutes. If you'd like the green onions to be more visible put them in the recipe at the very end. Make sure you use a good quality thick stainless steel pot so your chili does not burn on the bottom while it simmers, so you are not eating the ingredients your pot was made from or eating the residue from last week's dinner that had soaked into your pot.

Serve with a baked potato and salad topped with your favorite vinegar. My favorite is fig vinegar mixed with apple juice.

Spicy Tomato, Bean and Veggie Soup
1 box of organic low sodium vegetable broth
5 cups of filtered water
2 cups of cooked pinto beans not rinsed after cooking
1 extra-large can of crushed tomatoes
½ cup of chopped yellow onions
3 tbsp. fresh chopped jalapeño pepper
2 cups chopped baby carrots
1 cup chopped celery
1 cup diced zucchini
1 cup diced yellow squash
1 can washed organic corn
1 tsp. pink Himalayan salt
1 tsp. parsley
¼ tsp. pepper

The beauty of using already cooked beans is dinner is ready so much sooner! I try to have precooked beans in my fridge all the times to top salads, make the kids bean burritos, throw them in soft tacos or soups. If you have a pressure cooker you can cook beans much faster. If not, don't despair, just plan ahead! Soak you beans overnight, rinse and cook 30 minutes in a pressure cooker or 90 minutes in a soup pot. If needed, buy low sodium organic canned beans. We all have days when canned food is needed or very handy!

In a large stainless steel soup pot turn on medium heat and add vegetable broth, water, cooked pinto beans (warm or cold does not matter). You can use rinsed canned beans but it does not thicken as much as homemade beans still in a bit of bean juice. Cut out 1-2 cups of water if you are using canned beans. Add crushed tomatoes. While the soup is heating up chop and add your veggies, yellow onions, fresh chopped jalapeño pepper, carrots, celery, zucchini, yellow squash, and washed organic corn.

Season with pink Himalayan salt, parsley and pepper. Bring to a boil and then simmer for 20-30 minutes until the veggies are as soft as you like them. Enjoy with your favorite whole grain bread.

Sweet Potato Garbanzo Bean Soup
8 cups of filtered water
2 cups of washed and (soaked over-night if time permits) uncooked garbanzo beans
3 large sweet potatoes chopped in small pieces
1 cup chopped spinach
1 cup chopped celery
1 cup diced zucchini
1 cup diced yellow squash
1 bag organic frozen or thawed peas
1 tbsp. pink Himalayan salt
1 tbsp. garlic and herb seasoning
1 bay leaf
1 tsp. oregano

In a large stainless steel soup pot, turn the heat to medium and add 8 cups of filtered water, garbanzo beans and then chop and add to the soup while heating: sweet potatoes, spinach, celery, zucchini, yellow squash, frozen or thawed peas, pink Himalayan salt, garlic and herb seasoning, bay leaf (remove before serving) and oregano. Bring to a boil and then simmer on low heat for 90 minutes or until the beans are soft. If you are using cooked beans, simmer for 30 minutes only or until your veggies are as soft as you like them. Serve with your favorite whole grain bread.

Easy Quinoa Bean Salad
I love this recipe because it's so fast and easy! And you can make it in parts too. Cook the quinoa one day before, or earlier in the day, and chop and add the veggies later if you like.

101 THINGS I WISH I KNEW BEFORE I FED MY CHILDREN

2 cups quinoa cooked
1 can black beans
2 cups of any mix of veggies you like cooked or raw (frozen green peas and corn are great choices)
3 tomatoes
¼ cup diced green onions
1/3 cup apple cider vinegar
3 tbsp. honey
½ tsp. salt
½ tsp. pepper

This salad is so easy and so delicious and so versatile! You can even make it hot or cold. Start by washing and then cooking your quinoa. I prefer to chill the quinoa after I cook it so it's light and fluffy and less clumpy. Make sure to get a fine strainer that your quinoa won't slip through while you are washing it. Follow the quinoa cooking instructions on the bag. Quinoa gets sticky if you use too much water so be careful with your measuring. When I made the salad this time around, I cooked the quinoa on the stovetop and left in there for quite a few hours to cool. When we were ready for dinner I opened and washed one can of black beans (if you don't wash your beans the juice turns your salad dark and makes it not quite as pretty) and defrosted some corn and peas just until they were not frozen, and added them to the quinoa. I then chopped tomatoes from my garden, which I'm super excited about because it's winter and I have tomatoes! In years past I got tired of watering and weeding and let my garden go in the winter but this year I kept in going and was surprised it seemed to want to keep going with me! I then green onions from my window sill (when you buy green onions use them and save the stems and put them in water and re-grow in your kitchen window or replant in your garden. They seem to just keep producing!) Add apple cider vinegar, honey, salt and of pepper. Stir and enjoy!

Stuffing

I don't know about you, but stuffing is one of my very favorite holiday foods. Why save it for the holidays?

1 cup vegetable broth
½ cup diced yellow onions or ¼ cup green onions or both if you love onions!
1 cup chopped celery
1 loaf of fresh whole grain bread
2-3 cups of organic apple juice
1tsp. pink Himalayan salt
1tsp. dry parsley or a handful of fresh chopped parsley
1 tsp. of oregano or any of your favorite spices.

In an extra-large stainless steel sauce pan or medium size stainless soup pot, add your vegetable broth and turn the heat on to medium. Chop your onions and add to the simmering vegetable broth. Then do the same with your celery. Stir and let them simmer uncovered while you chop your loaf of bread into bite size pieces. The bread chopping should not take long. I break the sliced bread loaf into thirds and chop it with a large butcher knife, cutting it in fourths or fifths in each direction. Once the veggies are sautéed to your liking, add the chopped bread. Top with apple juice. We like the unfiltered apple juice. Apple juice is the secret ingredient that makes this recipe so sweet and delicious. Add your favorite spices. If you use more than two spices use ½ teaspoon instead of a full teaspoon of each or it might turn out too herby. Reduce the heat to low and stir for 3-5 minutes turning the bread to soak in the juices. We love to eat stuffing with potatoes or sweet potatoes and grilled veggies or salad. Grab a fork and enjoy!

White Bean Veggie Soup

1 bunch green onions chopped
1 tbsp. minced garlic

1 bag of white beans soak overnight or as long as you can
1 box organic low sodium veggie broth
8 cups water
1 chopped or spiralized zucchini
1 chopped or spiralized yellow squash
1 large can crushed tomatoes
1-2 tbsp. chopped fresh jalapeno-some like it hot!
Season to taste with your favorite herbs like salt, pepper, basil, parsley, thyme.
2 cups cooked rice

Turn the heat on your favorite stain steel pot and start adding ingredients. Add everything but the rice. Bring to a boil and simmer 1-2 hours until the beans are as tender as you like them. To make this recipe quicker, used canned beans and add those rinsed canned beans after the veggies are tender, or cook the beans in a pressure cooker while the soup heats and then add the soup to the beans, and you can be finished in 20 minutes. Once the soup is done, turn off the heat and add the cooked rice. Serve with your favorite whole grain bread. Delicious!

Veggie Burger
2 cups cooked brown rice
½ cup nutritional yeast
2 cans of your favorite beans washed and drained (I used 1 can of red kidney beans and one can of white northern beans)
¼ cup salsa
¼ cup barbecue sauce
1 tsp. onion powder
1 tsp. garlic powder

Mix all ingredients in a bowl and mash with a potato masher. Form patties by hand on throw on a hot nonstick skillet to warm and toast. Serve on your favorite 100% whole grain bread and top with your favorite burger toppings like mustard, caramelized onions, mushrooms, tomatoes and lettuce. Enjoy!

Cauliflower Scalloped Potatoes
I seem to come up with my best recipes when I have a shortage of ingredients and a lack of time, so I guess I should feel blessed about those things! Last night, time got away from me. There was only about 45 minutes until Ashley was leaving for dance class, so I needed to whip something up quick. I had red potatoes and cauliflower. I was thinking maybe some type of scalloped potatoes but I had never made a plant based scalloped potato dish and I was wondering if it could be any good without all the standard ingredients like cheese, cream soups and butter. The clock was ticking, so I went for it and it might just be one of our new favorites. I brought some to my daughter when I picked her up from lacrosse and she made me promise about 5 times that there was more waiting at home for her. Delicious!

2 cups organic oil-free low sodium vegetable broth, or make your own
1 tsp. minced garlic
½ cup chopped green onions
10 extra-large red potatoes, the size of your fist
1 large head of cauliflower
1 tsp. pink Himalayan salt
1/2 tsp. garlic powder
1 tsp. granulated onions
¼ tsp. pepper if you like some kick
* Optional— 2 tbsp. fresh chopped or dried minced parsley

Bread crumbs:
4 slices of bread
1/2 cup nutritional yeast
1/2 tsp. pink Himalayan salt

1 tsp. garlic powder
1 tsp. granulated onions

In an extra-large stainless steel pot, turn on medium heat and add the vegetable broth, minced garlic and chopped green onions. (You should only have to buy green onions a few times. Once you use them replant the left over stalk in either a cup of water in your window or in a little pot outside. They grow back in less than 2 weeks and you can just keep chopping and enjoying. While that is heating up wash and run the potatoes through a food processor with a slicing blade so the slices are around 1/8th inch thick and pour them into the simmering pot. Next wash and run the cauliflower through the food processor with the same blade and then add those to the stovetop. Add your seasonings and stir. Cover and simmer for 30 minutes stirring every 10 minutes or so. If it gets too dry, add a bit more vegetable broth. While the scalloped potatoes finish cooking, throw some bread in the food processor with a chopping blade to make some bread crumbs. Add the seasoning and chop until they turn to crumbs. Once the potatoes are soft, sprinkle with bread crumbs and serve. You'll have extra bread crumbs so set them out for those who love bread crumbs and want to add more. Here's to your health!

Yammy Lasagna
Lasagna has always been a favorite of mine, but how do you enjoy it without cheese? I've been playing with different recipes and have come up with one I love. It's my very yummy lasagna! I hope you enjoy it as much as I do. It is a bit labor intensive, so be sure to make it when you are not in a rush to get dinner on the table. Bean burritos are great for those rushed nights! As always, I make huge servings for my family of six, plus enough to share with others and eat leftovers the next day. Shrink this recipe in half if you are not feeding an army like I tend to.

3 zucchinis
3 yellow squashes

*mushrooms (optional veggie addition)
½ cup green onions
1 cup water
1 tsp. Himalayan salt
1 tsp. onion powder
1 tsp. garlic powder
1 tbsp. Italian seasoning
1 10 oz. box of lasagna noodles
3 jars of oil free (fat free) pasta sauce
4 baked yams
4 tomatoes
1 cup nutritional yeast

Chop and stir fry zucchinis, yellow squashes, mushrooms (optional veggie addition), green onions, water, Himalayan salt, onion powder and garlic powder. Once the veggies are cooked, set them aside and start building your lasagna. Use an oversized glass casserole dish (12x15). Pour ¾ of the jar of pasta sauce in the bottom of the pan, then cover the sauce with noodles. Next, top the noodles with the stir fried veggies, top with another layer of sauce (enough to cover the veggies), and then with another layer of noodles. Peel and mash your yams and spread them on top of the noodles. Next, cover with a layer of pasta sauce. Slice your tomatoes thick and cover the top of the lasagna with them. Sprinkle nutritional yeast over the top. Cover with parchment paper and then foil. Bake for 1 hour at 350 degrees. Uncover and bake for an additional 15 minutes. Serve with a side salad and bread, or over a bed of spinach. So yummy!

Spaghetti
Here is a quick and easy dinner that should keep everyone happy! Who does not love spaghetti? This is a meal I cook for company and when kids have friends over. It's fast, cheap and delicious.

1 bag whole grain spaghetti
1 jar oil free pasta sauce
1-2 tbsp. nutritional yeast
8 slices of whole grain bread
1/4 cup spreadable cashew cheese
1 tsp. of garlic granules

Cook the pasta as instructed on the package. Our favorite pasta is brown rice pasta. Strain and rinse with hot water. Fight the urge to pour olive oil on it after you strain it. I know you want to! Top with an oil free marinara sauce. For those who like it, sprinkle with nutritional yeast which has a nutty, cheesy flavor. While the pasta is cooking, put your oven on high broil. Spread 8 slices of bread with homemade cashew cheese and sprinkle with garlic granules. Broil for 3-5 minutes. Don't let the bread burn! Serve with a fresh green salad and steamed broccoli or green peas.

DESSERT

No-Bake Strawberry Pie
1½ cup walnuts
1½ cup pitted dates + 8 more dates
1 tsp. vanilla
2 pts fresh strawberries
½ tsp. lemon juice

For the crust, add walnuts, 1½ cups of pitted dates, and vanilla and chop in a food processor for about 45 seconds, then press into the pie pan for the crust. Next, puree the strawberries and the 8 dates in the processor with the lemon until blended smooth and pour into the crust. Next, slice more strawberries and top your pie with them. Refrigerate for two hours so it has time to set up and slice like a pie. It won't be 100% sliceable but close. If you can't wait for the cooling, grab a spoon and dig in! If you are using a larger pie pan, double the recipe. My neighbor loved the crust so much that she rolled it into little balls dusted with flour (or you could use coconut), and served as a treat for her kids. So smart!

Chocolate Milk Shake
2 cups of your favorite non-dairy milk
4 frozen ripe sliced bananas
4 tbsp. cocoa powder
1 tsp. vanilla

Blend in a high power blender and enjoy!

Vanilla Milk Shake
2 cups of your favorite non-dairy milk
4 chopped frozen bananas
1 tsp. vanilla

Blend in a high power blender and enjoy!

Strawberry Milk Shake
2 cups coconut milk
2 cups chopped frozen bananas
2 cups chopped frozen strawberries
1 tsp. vanilla

Blend in a high power blender and enjoy!

Fruit Salad
We love having fruit salad for dessert! Chop any fresh fruit you have, mix and enjoy! You can sprinkle with chopped nuts, coconut and even a drizzle of maple syrup if you want it even sweeter.

Apple Cake
This is a Chef Brad recipe that I love! I edited it to make it plant based. It's just as yummy as ever!

3 to 4 large baking apples, pealed
1 cup applesauce
1 cup 100% pure organic maple syrup
Ener-g egg replacer to replace 4 eggs
1 cup non-dairy milk
2 tsp. vanilla
3 ½ cups fresh ground spelt flour
1 tbsp. baking powder
1 tsp. pumpkin pie spice
1 tsp. dried chipotle chili powder
1 tsp. pink salt
*optional—add one cup of chopped walnuts

Wondering what to do with all those apples that are getting a bit to mushy to eat? Don't let them go to waste! Time to make an apple cake! Grate apples on a fine grater or run them through the food processor on a grating blade. Remove seeds and core first! Put applesauce, syrup, egg replacer, and vanilla in the blender and whip. Add the whipped ingredients to flour and additional ingredients and mix. Pour into a 12x15" glass baking pan. In a preheated oven, bake at 350 degrees for 35 to 45 minutes. Top with fresh fruit and enjoy!

FIND JENNY

For my latest health tips and recipes, follow me at:
www.NourishAndStrengthen.org
And on Facebook @ Nourish and Strengthen.
Emails to Jenny@NourishAndStrengthen.org

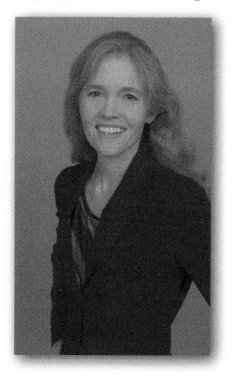

ABOUT THE AUTHOR

Jenny Harkleroad was born on in Laguna Beach, CA and has lived in San Diego County since she was 3. Jenny is the oldest of three children. She grew up a typical overachiever in school, sports and music. Jenny is married to her high school sweetheart and they have 4 spectacular children.

After over a decade in a fast paced and successful real estate career, Jenny broke her back in a hiking accident. With a lot of down time during her recovery, she began looking at her life, and realized she hadn't been living authentically. Her curiosity, introspection and health trouble led to many new passions including plant-based eating, healthier cooking, gardening, teaching, writing, blogging and studying ways to help the body and mind succeed physically, mentally, emotionally, and spiritually.

Jenny now runs a business helping others change self-limiting subconscious beliefs. This method helps people quickly accomplish all their goals including eating healthy. When the subconscious is on board, it's amazing what can happen!

Jenny has a strong belief in God and appreciates His hand in her life and is grateful to see it every day. Jenny is excited about her new found love of health. She never knew what a difference eating well could make until she faced and cured (with the help of others) her own health challenges. Jenny hopes to pass this life saving information on to you and your families. Here's to your health!

NOTES

1. How To Eat Right In the Real World by Robyn Oppenshaw, http://greensmoothiegirl.com/product/nutrition/how-to-eat-right-in-the-real-world/.

2. Fusion Grain Cooking on BYUtv by Chef Brad, http://www.byutv.org/show/6ef10280-3ab2-42f0-9431-8c3ff800d794/chef-brad-fusion-grain-cooking.

3. The Doctrine and Covenants Section 89 by Joseph Smith, https://www.lds.org/scriptures/dc-testament/dc/89?lang=eng.

4. The China Study by T. Colin Campbell, PhD & Thomas M. Campbell II, 2006, p. 13 and p. 55.

5. The China Study by T. Colin Campbell, PhD & Thomas M. Campbell II, 2006, p. 15.

6. Prevent and Reverse Heart Disease, Caldwell Esselstyn Jr. M.D., 2007.

7. Prevent and Reverse Heart Disease, Caldwell Esselstyn Jr. M.D., 2007, p. 1.

8. American Cancer Society, www.cancer.org.

9. Cancer Facts and Figures 2016, American Cancer Society, http://www.cancer.org/acs/groups/content/@research/documents/document/acspc-047079.pdf.

10. Cancer Facts and Figures 2016, American Cancer Society, http://www.cancer.org/acs/groups/content/@research/documents/document/acspc-047079.pdf.

11. Cancer Facts and Figures 2015, American Cancer Society, http://www.cancer.org/acs/groups/content/@editorial/documents/document/acspc-044552.pdf.

12. The China Study, T. Colin Campbell, PhD and Thomas M. Campbell II, 2006 p. 15.

13. Dr. John McDougall, *"Diabetes, Drugs and 100 Years of Missed Opportunities"* https://www.drmcdougall.com/health/education/videos/free-electures/diet-drugs-and-diabetes/.

14. The China Study, T. Colin Campbell, PhD and Thomas M. Campbell II, 2006 p. 15.

15. The Starch Solution, John A. McDougall, MD, 2012 Page 10.

16. The Starch Solution, John A. McDougall, MD, 2012 p. 9.

17. Wikipedia, https://en.wikipedia.org/wiki/Legume.

18. The Starch Solution, John A. McDougall, MD, 2012 p. 13.

19. The China Study by T. Colin Campbell, PhD & Thomas M. Campbell II, 2006, p. 27-38.

20. The China Study by T. Colin Campbell, PhD & Thomas M. Campbell II, 2006, p. 28.

21. Grains with the Highest Protein to Carbohydrate Ratio, Daisy Whitbread, certified nutritionist and Paul House, health analyst, http://www.healthaliciousness.com/articles/grains-highest-protein-carbohydrate-ratio.php.

22. 37 Beans and Legumes with the Most Protein, Daisy Whitbread, certified nutritionist and Paul House, health analyst, http://www.healthaliciousness.com/articles/beans-legumes-highest-protein.php.

23. 27 Vegetables Highest in Protein, Daisy Whitbread, certified nutritionist and Paul House, health analyst, http://www.healthaliciousness.com/articles/vegetables-high-in-protein.php.

24. 23 Fruits Highest in Protein, Daisy Whitbread, certified nutritionist and Paul House, health analyst, http://www.healthaliciousness.com/articles/fruits-high-in-protein.php.

25. The China Study by T. Colin Campbell, PhD & Thomas M. Campbell II, 2006, p. 31.

26. Mr. Universe Goes Vegan, Joshua Katcher, July 14, 2015, http://thediscerningbrute.com/mr-universe-goes-vegan/.

27. Patrik Baboumian, Vegan Strongman, http://www.greatveganathletes.com/patrik-baboumian-vegan-strongman.

28. Rich Roll 201 Podcast, https://soundcloud.com/richroll/rrp201.

29. What You Can Do to Help Farmed Animals, Free From Harm Staff Writers, January 4, 2010, Mclanie Joy, Social Psychologist, http://freefromharm.org/what-you-can-do-to-help-farm-animals/.

30. For the Love of Grains, John McDougall MD, McDougall Newsletter, January 2008, https://www.drmcdougall.com/misc/2008nl/jan/grains.htm.

31. High Protein Diets, John McDougall MD, https://www.drmcdougall.com/health/education/health-science/featured-articles/articles/high-protein-diets/.

32. 15 Reasons Why You May Want To Reconsider Eating Meat, Evita Ochel, April 18, 2009, updated April 1, 2016, http://www.evolvingwellness.com/essay/15-reasons-why-you-may-want-to-reconsider-eating-meat.

33. Vitamin B12 Deficiency, Not Just for Vegans Anymore! http://bitesizevegan.com/vegan-health/vitamin-b12-deficiency-not-just-for-vegans-anymore/.

34. Researchers Find Evidence of Banned Antibiotics in Poultry Products, Johns Hopkins, Bloomberg School of Public Health, April 5, 2012. http://www.jhsph.edu/news/news-releases/2012/feather-meal-clf.html.

35. Discovering The Word Of Wisdom, Jane Birch, 2013, p. 40.

36. Prevent and Reverse Heart Disease, Caldwell Esselstyn Jr. M.D., 2007.

37. It's The Food!, The McDougall Blog, https://www.drmcdougall.com/connections/its-the-food/.

38. McDougall Advanced Study Weekend, February 12-14, 2016, Dr. Scott Stoll.

39. The China Study by T. Colin Campbell, PhD & Thomas M. Campbell II, 2006 p. 71.

40. 12 Frightening Facts About Milk, Thomas Campbell, MD, October 31, 2014 http://nutritionstudies.org/12-frightening-facts-milk/.

41. Calcium in Plant-Based Diets, Physicians Committee for Responsible Medicine, http://www.pcrm.org/health/diets/vsk/vegetarian-starter-kit-calcium.

42. Calcium-Where do I get Calcium, Dr. Esselstyns Prevent and Reverse Heart Disease Program, http://www.dresselstyn.com/site/faq/.

43. Whole Food Plant-Based (WFPB) Guidelines, Jane Birch, http://discoveringthewordofwisdom.com/wfpb-guidelines/.

44. Your Heart On Plants, Dr. Robert Ostfeld, Cardiologist, McDougall Advanced Study Weekend February 12-14, 2016.

45. Dr. Caldwell Esselstyn, McDougall Advanced Study Weekend February 12-14, 2016.

46. Dr. Caldwell Esselstyn, McDougall Advanced Study Weekend February 12-14, 2016.

47. Fish Oil-Should I take fish oil? FAQ, Dr. Esselstyn's Prevent and Reverse Heart Disease Program, http://www.dresselstyn.com/site/faq/.

48. Vegetarians Make Plenty of Essential Fats (DHA), My Favorite Five from Recent Medical Journals, McDougall Newsletter, Dr. John McDougall, September 2009, https://www.drmcdougall.com/misc/2009nl/sep/fav5.htm.

49. To Take or Not To Take Fish Oil, T. Colin Campbell, PhD, December 15, 2009, Modified November 16, 2015, http://nutritionstudies.org/to-take-or-not-to-take-fish-oil/.

50. Confessions of a Fish Killer, McDougall Newsletter, John McDougall, MD, June 2007, https://www.drmcdougall.com/misc/2007nl/jun/confessions.htm.

51. Dr. McDougall's Health & Medical Center, www.Dr.McDougall.com.

52. The Egg Industry: Exposing a Source of Food Poisoning, It's the Food, The McDougall Newsletter, John McDougall MD, January 2016, https://www.drmcdougall.com/misc/2016nl/jan/eggindustry.htm.

53. Lies and Damned Lies: Damned Lies Harm the Public and Planet Earth, It's the Food, The McDougall Newsletter, John McDougall MD, June 2015 https://www.drmcdougall.com/misc/2015nl/jun/lies.htm.

54. Dietary Guidelines-Previous Guidelines, United States Department of Agriculture, Center for Nutrition Policy and Promotion, http://www.cnpp.usda.gov/dietary-guidelines-previous-guidelines.

55. Physicians Committee for Responsible Medicine, http://www.pcrm.org/.

56. The McDougall Plan, John McDougall MD, October 22, 1983, https://www.drmcdougall.com/health/shopping/ebooks/mcdougall-plan/.

57. Dietary cholesterol from eggs increases the ratio of total cholesterol to high-density lipoprotein cholesterol in humans: a meta-analysis, Rianne M. Weggman, Peter L. Zock, and Martijn B. Katan, The American Journal of Clinical Nutrition, 2001, http://ajcn.nutrition.org/content/73/5/885.full.pdf+html.

58. The Oxford Vegetarian Study: an Overview 1'2'3', Paul N Appleby, Margaret Thorogood, Jim I. Mann, and Timothy JA Key, 1999 American Society for Clinical Nutrition, The American Journal of Clinical Nutrition, http://ajcn.nutrition.org/content/70/3/525s.ful.

59. Dietary Cholesterol and Plasma Lipoprotein Profiles: Randomized Controlled Trials, John D. Griffin, M.S. and Alice H. Lichtenstein, D. Sc., National Institute of Health, NIH Public Access Author Manuscript, December 2013, http://www.ncbi.nlm.nih.gov/pmc/articles/PMC3900007/pdf/nihms532744.pdf.

60. Eggs, Michael Greger M.D., August 8, 2016, http://nutritionfacts.org/topics/eggs/.

61. Starch Staples, Dr. McDougall Health & Medical Center, https://www.drmcdougall.com/health/education/free-mcdougall-program/steps-to-recovery/starch-staples/.

62. How To Eat Right in the Real World, Robyn Oppenshaw, p. 8.

63. Keeping It Simple On A Whole Foods Plants-Based Diet, Holly, January 26, 2015, http://myplantbasedfamily.com/2015/01/26/keeping-simple-whole-foods-plant-based-diet/.

64. Food Poisoning, How to cure it by eating beans, corn, pasta, potatoes, rice, etc., Dr. McDougall's Color Picture Book, https://www.drmcdougall.com/wp/wp-content/uploads/Dr.-McDougalls-Color-Picture-Book1.pdf.

65. The China Study by T. Colin Campbell, PhD & Thomas M. Campbell II, 2006, p. 54-67.

66. The China Study by T. Colin Campbell, PhD & Thomas M. Campbell II, 2006, p. 204-211.

67. The Starch Solution, John A. McDougall, MD, 2012 p.142-145.

68. Vegetable Fats As Medicine, Greater Risks of Heart Disease, John McDougall, MD, https://www.drmcdougall.com/health/education/health-science/featured-articles/articles/vegetable-fat-as-medicine/.

69. Cowspiracy, The Sustainability Secret, The Facts, http://www.cowspiracy.com/infographic.

70. Scarcity vs. Distribution, Exporting Foods as Distribution, A Well-Fed World, Feeding Families/Saving Animals, http://awfw.org/scarcity-vs-distribution/.

71. Whole, T. Colin Campbell, PhD with Howard Jacobson, PhD, 2013, p. 96.

72. The China Study, T. Colin Campbell, PhD & Thomas M. Campbell II, 2006, p. 48-67.

73. Different Words for Sugar on Food Labels, Elizabeth Brown, http://healthyeating.sfgate.com/different-words-sugar-food-labels-8373.html.

74. Diabetes, drugs and 100 years of missed opportunities, John McDougall MD, Advanced Study Weekend, Santa Rosa CA, https://www.drmcdougall.com/health/education/videos/free-electures/diet-drugs-and-diabetes/.

75. Plant-Based On A Budget: Strategies For Affordable Cooking And Eating, Micaela Karlsen, MSPH, August 8, 2016, http://www.forksoverknives.com/plant-based-budget-strategies-affordable-cooking-eating/.

76. McDougall Advanced Study Weekend, February 12-14th, 2016 in Santa Rosa California. I purchased and watched a recording of the event online.

77. The Benefits of Himalayan Salt, Dr. Edward Group, May 15, 2009, updated July 31, 2014, http://www.globalhealingcenter.com/natural-health/Himalayan-crystal-salt-benefits/.

78. Fat Free Vegan Kitchen, Susan Voisin, http://blog.fatfreevegan.com/category/desserts.

79. The China Study by T. Colin Campbell, PhD & Thomas M. Campbell II, 2006, p.48-67.

80. The China Study by T. Colin Campbell, PhD & Thomas M. Campbell II, 2006, p.69-108.

81. The China Study by T. Colin Campbell, PhD & Thomas M. Campbell II, 2006, p.48-67.

82. The Starch Solution, John A. McDougall, MD, 2012.

83. In Cholesterol Lowering, Moderation Kills, Caldwell B. Esselstyn Jr. MD, Department of General Surgery, Cleveland Clinic Foundation,

Caldwell Esselstyn Jr. M.D., Prevent and Reverse Heart Disease, 2007.

84. Heart Disease: A Toothless Paper Tiger That Need Never Exist, Kathy Freston, March 18, 2010 updated November 17, 2011, http://www.huffingtonpost.com/kathy-freston/heart-disease-a-toothless_b_334285.html.

85. The Smoke and Mirrors behind Wheat Belly and Grain Brain, Dr. McDougall's Health & Medical Center, January 2014 Newsletter, https://www.drmcdougall.com/misc/2014nl/jan/smoke.htm.

86. The China Study by T. Colin Campbell, PhD & Thomas M. Campbell II, 2006.

87. Prevent and Reverse Heart Disease, Caldwell Esselstyn Jr. M.D., 2007.

88. The Starch Solution, John A. McDougall, MD, 2012.

89. Dr. McDougall's Health & Medical Center, https://www.drmcdougall.com/.

90. Man In The Mirror, Michael Jackson, https://en.wikipedia.org/wiki/Man_in_the_Mirror.

91. Cowspiracy, The Sustainability Secret, http://www.cowspiracy.com/.

92. Antiobiotics, Grace Communication Foundation, http://www.sustainabletable.org/257/antibiotics.

93. Pesticides, Grace Communication Foundation, http://www.sustainabletable.org/263/pesticides.

94. Additives, Grace Communication Foundation, http://www.sustainabletable.org/385/additives.

95. Hormones, Grace Communication Foundation, http://www.sustainabletable.org/258/hormones.

96. Welfare, Grace Communication Foundation, http://www.sustainabletable.org/274/animal-welfare.

97. Bjelakovic G., Nikolova D., Gluud L.L., Simonetti R.G., Gluud C. Mortality in Randomized Trials of Antioxidant Supplements for Primary and Secondary Prevention: Systematic Review and Meta-analysis. *JAMA*. 2007 Feb 28;297(8):842-57, http://www.ncbi.nlm.nih.gov/pubmed/17327526.

98. Vitamin D Supplements Are Harmful-Sunshine and Food Determine Health, Dr. John McDougall, MD, March 2015 Newsletter, https://www.drmcdougall.com/misc/2015nl/mar/vitamind.htm.

99. Just To Be On The Safe Side: Don't Take Vitamins, Dr. John McDougall, May 2010 Newsletter, https://www.drmcdougall.com/misc/2010nl/may/100500.htm.

100. I Say "No" to Flu Vaccines, Dr. John McDougall, M.D., November 2014 Newsletter, https://www.drmcdougall.com/misc/2014nl/nov/flushot.htm.

101. https://www.drmcdougall.com/misc/2014nl/nov/flushot.htm.

102. Dr. Robert W. Sears M.D., FAAP, The Vaccine Book, 2011.

103. The Vaccine Book, Dr. Robert W. Sears M.D, www.thevaccine-book.com.

104. www.facebook.com/dr-bob-sears.

105. Drinking Water In The Morning, New Health Guide, http://www.newhealthguide.org/Drinking-Water-In-The-Morning.html.

106. Compelling Facts, The Plantrician Project, www.Plantricianproject.com.

107. The China Study, Wikipedia, https://en.wikipedia.org/wiki/The_China_Study.

108. Pinterest Vegetable Trays, https://www.pinterest.com/explore/vegetable-trays/.

109. Prevent and Reverse Heart Disease, Caldwell Esselstyn Jr. M.D., 2007.

110. Dr. Esselstyn's Prevent & Reverse Heart Disease Program, http://www.dresselstyn.com/site/faq.

111. Disease-Proof Your Child, Dr. Joel Fuhrman M.D., 2005.

112. Disease-Proof Your Child, Dr. Joel Fuhrman M.D., 2005, p. 48-49.

113. Disease-Proof Your Child, Dr. Joel Fuhrman M.D., 2005, p. 50.

114. Disease-Proof Your Child, Dr. Joel Fuhrman M.D., 2005, p. 53.

115. Disease-Proof Your Child, Dr. Joel Fuhrman M.D., 2005, p. 54.

116. Disease-Proof Your Child, Dr. Joel Fuhrman M.D., 2005, p. 55.

117. Disease-Proof Your Child, Dr. Joel Fuhrman M.D., 2005, p. 56-57.

118. EWG's 2016 Shopper's Guide to Pesticides in Produce™, https://www.ewg.org/foodnews/summary.php.

119. Chef Brad's WonderFlour, http://chefbrad.com/2016/06/chef-brads-wonderflour/.

120. Simple Daily Recipes, Jill McKeever, https://www.youtube.com/user/SimpleDailyRecipes.

121. Nourish and Strengthen, http://nourishandstrengthen.org/.

122. Facebook, Nourish and Strengthen, https://www.facebook.com/NourishAndStrengthen/.

123. The Starch Solution "Secrets", John McDougall M.D., January 7, 2016, https://www.drmcdougall.com/health/education/webinars/webinar-1-7-16/.

124. Blue Zones Live Longer, Better, Dan Buettner, https://www.bluezones.com/resources/books/.

125. Color Picture Book, John McDougall M.D., https://www.drmcdougall.com/health/education/cpb/.

126. McDougall Newsletter Recipes, https://www.drmcdougall.com/health/education/recipes/mcdougall-newsletter-recipes/.

127. Sugar, Coated With Myths, John McDougall MD, September 2006, https://www.drmcdougall.com/misc/2006nl/sept/sugar.htm.

128. The Dietary Guidelines for 2015-2020, John McDougall M.D., https://www.drmcdougall.com/health/education/webinars/webinar-03-03-16/.

129. United States District Court, Northern District of California, Physicians Committee for Responsible Medicine, John McDougall MD, Ulka Agarwal MD, Debra Shapino MD, Ulka Agarwal MD, Debra Shapino MD, plantiffs v. Thomas Vilsack, Secretary United States Department of Agriculture and Sylvia Mathews Burwell, Secretary, Department of Health and Human Services, defendants, https://www.drmcdougall.com/misc/2016nl/jan/lawsuitdgac.pdf.

130. Walter Kempner, MD, Founder Of The Rice Diet, McDougall December 2013 Newsletter, John McDougall, MD, https://www.drmcdougall.com/2013/12/31/walter-kempner-md-founder-of-the-rice-diet/.

131. The China Study, T. Colin Campbell, PhD & Thomas M. Campbell II, 2006.

132. Why You Simply MUST Filter Your Water, Dr. Frank Lipman, April 4, 2014, http://www.mindbodygreen.com/0-13217/why-you-simply-must-filter-your-water.html.

133. Health Benefits of Sprouts, https://www.organicfacts.net/health-benefits/seed-and-nut/sprouts.html.

134. Family Movie Night, Jenny Harkleroad, May 23, 2016 http://nourishandstrengthen.org/family-movie-night/.

135. Understanding Food Dye Allergies, Stephanie Watson, Medically Reviewed by Steven Kim MD, June 25, 2015, http://www.healthline.com/health/allergies/understanding-food-dye-allergies#Overview1.

136. *Grown Ups*, 2010, https://www.youtube.com/watch?v=wVsMJ0ntvmc.

137. Infants And Allergies: What Parents Should Watch For, Chris Iliades, MD, Medically Reviewed By Pat F. Bass III MD, MS, MPH. http://www.everydayhealth.com/allergy/infants-and-allergies-what-should-parents-watch-for.aspx.

138. Milk Allergy, http://www.mayoclinic.org/diseases-conditions/milk-allergy/basics/symptoms/con-20032147.

139. Appetizers And Dips, FatFree Vegan Kitchen, Susan Voisin, http://blog.fatfreevegan.com/category/appetizers-and-dips.

140. Chef Ann Foundation. Changing The Way We Feed Our Kids, http://www.chefannfoundation.org/.

141. Can't Be Beet Chocolate Cake! Fat Free Vegan Kitchen, Susan Voisin, February 28, 2006, http://blog.fatfreevegan.com/2006/02/cant-be-beet-chocolate-cake.html.

142. The Doctrine and Covenants, Section 89:1-21, Joseph Smith, February 27, 1833, https://www.lds.org/scriptures/dc-testament/dc/89?lang=eng.

143. Chef Brad, America's Grain Guy, www.ChefBrad.com.

144. The Fat You Eat, Is The Fat You Wear, John McDougall MD, 2/25/16. https://www.youtube.com/watch?v=-KBicWwnCdg.

145. People Passionate About Starches Are Healthy And Beautiful People, John McDougall MD, March 2009, https://www.drmcdougall.com/misc/2009nl/mar/passionate.htm.

146. Prevent and Reverse Heart Disease, Caldwell Esselstyn Jr. M.D., 2007, p. 35-45.

147. Jenny Harkleroad, Balanced You, www.BalancedYou.org.

148. Dr. McDougall's Color Picture Book, John McDougall MD, https://www.drmcdougall.com/health/education/cpb/.

149. Vitamin B12: Are You Getting It? Jack Norris, Registered Dietitian, http://www.veganhealth.org/articles/vitaminb12.

150. William Ripple, PhD: Environmental Effects of Human Carvinory, McDougall Advanced Study Weekend, February 2016, McDougall Advanced Study Weekend, February 2016.

151. Prevent and Reverse Heart Disease, Caldwell Esselstyn Jr. M.D., 2007, p. 38.

152. Shark Killing Is Down 50% Thanks to Yao Ming, October 22, 2015. https://www.youtube.com/watch?v=NJZADv9wuGs.

153. Forks Over Knives, Virgil Films, September 8, 2011. https://www.youtube.com/watch?v=DZb-35oV_7E.

154. The Widowmaker, http://widowmakerthemovie.com/.

155. Cowspiracy, The Sustainability Secret, A.U.M. Films & First Spark Media, Kip Andersen & Keegan Kuhn, 2014 http://www.cowspiracy.com/.

156. Plant Pure Nation, July 4, 2015, https://www.youtube.com/watch?v=9E6sa0OtjSE.

157. Back To Eden, https://vimeo.com/28055108.

158. Taking Life, Steve Reed, August 27, 2016, http://discoveringthewordofwisdom.com/wow-reflections-steve-reed/#more-3926.

159. The Plantrician Project, Planting Seeds of Change, http://plantricianproject.org/.

160. Guess What? You're Buying Fake Maple Syrup! Tamara Mannelly, http://ohlardy.com/guess-what-youre-eating-fake-maple-syrup/.

161. GreenSmoothieGirl: Making Organic Fresh Salsa In Five Minutes, July 23, 2009, https://www.youtube.com/watch?v=qJnlgoomU5M.

162. For The Love of Grains, John McDougall MD, January 2008, https://www.drmcdougall.com/misc/2008nl/jan/grains.pdf.

163. Just A Little More About Starch and The Starch Solution, John McDougall MD, July 2011, https://www.drmcdougall.com/misc/2012nl/feb/excerpt.htm.

164. Montefiore Doing More, Robert J. Ostfeld, MD, MS, http://www.montefiore.org/body.cfm?id=1735&action=detail&ref=729.

165. Advice From A Vegan Cardiologist, Dr. Kim A. Williams, President elect of the American College of Cardiology, The New York Times, August 6th, 2014, http://well.blogs.nytimes.com/2014/08/06/advice-from-a-vegan-cardiologist/.

166. The Smoke and Mirrors Behind Wheat Belly and Grain Brain, John McDougall MD, January 2014, https://www.drmcdougall.com/misc/2014nl/jan/smoke.htm.

167. Obesity, John McDougall MD, https://www.drmcdougall.com/health/education/health-science/common-health-problems/obesity/.

168. What The Heck Is Nutritional Yeast? Susan Voisin, October 26, 2011, http://blog.fatfreevegan.com/2011/10/what-the-heck-is-nutritional-yeast.html.

169. Chef Brad's WonderFlour, http://chefbrad.com/category/recipes/wonderflour-recipes/.

170. 10 Tips From A Pediatrician: How To Feed Your Plant-Based Family Without Losing Your Mind, Reshma Shad, MD, July 27, 2016, http://www.forksoverknives.com/10-tips-pediatrician-feed-plant-based-family-without-losing-mind/.

171. What Forcing Kids To Eat Look Like 20 Years Later, Maryann Tomovich Jacobson, MS, RD On July 6, 2012, http://www.raisehealthyeaters.com/2012/07/what-forcing-kids-to-eat-looks-like-20-years-later/.

172. The Five Secrets of Effective Communication, David D. Burns, http://helpingmarriageswork.com/docs/resources/the-five-secrets-of-effective-communication.pdf?sfvrsn=3.

173. Feeling Good Together: The Secret To Making Troubled Relationships Work, David D. Burns, M.D., http://www.goodreads.com/book/show/5680626-feeling-good-together.

174. Looking for a Plant-Based Doc? The Plantrician Project, http://plantricianproject.org/plant-based-docs.

175. Prevent and Reverse Heart Disease, Caldwell Esselstyn Jr. M.D., 2007.

176. Cowspiracy, The Sustainability Secret, http://www.cowspiracy.com/.

177. Talk of the Town: Burgers v. Oprah, The New York Times, Sam Howe Verhovek, January 21, 1998, http://www.nytimes.com/1998/01/21/us/talk-of-the-town-burgers-v-oprah.html.

178. HOMEMADE RAW DATE SYRUP, Zoe Tattersall, December 21, 2012, http://zomt.com.au/2012/12/homemade-raw-date-syrup.html.

179. Homemade Date Paste, The Ultimate All Natural Sweetener, Deborah Mele, 2014, http://www.italianfoodforever.com/2014/11/homemade-date-paste/.

180. Experts Know-Drug Companies Buy Research And Medical Journals, John McDougall MD, June 2005, https://www.drmcdougall.com/misc/2005nl/june/050600richardsmith.htm.

181. Color Your World With Fruits And Vegetables, Andrea Donsky, http://naturallysavvy.com/eat/color-your-world.

182. 7 Keys To Success On A Healthy Vegan Diet, Brian Wendel, July 20, 2016, http://www.forksoverknives.com/7-tips-succeed-healthy-vegan-diet/.

183. Eat When Hungry-Stop When Satisfied, Caryn Honig, MEd, RD, LD, http://www.thehealthyweighonline.com/eat-when-hungry-stop-when-satisfied/.

184. Your Guide To Soaking & Sprouting Whole Grains, Beans, Nuts, & Seeds, Danelle Wolford, http://www.weedemandreap.com/guide-soaking-sprouting-grains/.

185. Kitchen Scraps You Can Regrow With Nothing But Water, Thorin Klosowski, February 26, 2014, http://lifehacker.com/kitchen-scraps-you-can-regrow-with-nothing-but-water-1531011995.

186. Soy, Food, Wonder Drug, or Poison? John McDougall MD, April 2005, https://www.drmcdougall.com/misc/2005nl/april/050400pusoy.htm.

187. Pharmed Out Bios, Who We Are, http://pharmedout.org/bios.html.

188. About Glycemic Index, The University of Sydney, Last Updated May 3, 2016, http://www.glycemicindex.com/about.php.

189. http://www.glycemicindex.com/about.php.

190. 20 Healthiest Spices on Earth, http://bembu.com/healthy-spices-and-herbs.

191. Smoking, Michael Greger M.D., Last Updated August 4th, 2016, http://nutritionfacts.org/topics/smoking/.

192. Nutrition Facts, Michael Greger M.D http://nutritionfacts.org/.

193. American Medical Association Complicity With Big Tobacco, Michael Greger M.D., June 22, 2016, http://nutritionfacts.org/video/american-medical-association-complicity-big-tobacco/.

194. Nutrition Facts, Michael Greger M.D http://nutritionfacts.org/.

195. McDougall Advanced Study Weekend February 2016.

196. McDougall Advanced Study Weekend February 2016.

197. 2 Kings 5:1-14, Old Testament, King James Bible, https://www.lds.org/search?q=2+kings+5%3a1-14&lang=eng&domains=scriptures.

198. Effect of Chocolate On Acne Vulgaris, Fulton JE Jr. *JAMA*. 1969 Dec. 15;210(11):2071-4.

199. Acne Has Nothing To Do With Diet-Wrong!, John McDougall MD, November 2003, https://www.drmcdougall.com/misc/2003nl/nov/acne.htm.

200. Track Your Progress, John McDougall MD, https://www.drmcdougall.com/health/education/free-mcdougall-program/steps-to-recovery/track-your-progress/.

201. www.KelliRussell.com

202. www.yogaboost.co

203. McDougall Advanced Study Weekend, February 2016.

204. Comfortably Unaware, Dr. Richard A. Oppenlander, 2012, http://comfortablyunaware.com/.

205. Comfortably Unaware, Dr. Richard A. Oppenlander, 2012, http://comfortablyunaware.com/.

206. The Benefits of Organic Shampoo and Conditioners, Dr. Edward Group DC, NP, DACBN, DABFM, January 12, 2016, http://www.globalhealingcenter.com/natural-health/benefits-of-organic-shampoo-and-conditioners/.

207. The Benefits of Organic Laundry Detergent, Dr. Edward Group DC, NP, DACBN, DABFM, June 24, 2014, http://www.globalhealingcenter.com/natural-health/the-benefits-of-organic-laundry-detergent/.

208. Why You Should Use Natural Deodorant, Gina Debacker, July/August 2014, http://www.motherearthliving.com/health-and-wellness/natural-beauty/natural-deodorant-zmez14jazpit.aspx.

209. EWG's Guide To Healthy Cleaning, http://www.ewg.org/guides/cleaners.

210. A Step-By-Step Guide To Dry Skin Brushing, Olivia Jenkins, February 19, 2014, http://www.mindbodygreen.com/0-12675/a-step-by-step-guide-to-dry-skin-brushing.html.

211. Joanie Greggains—Workouts, http://www.joaniegreggains.com/dvdscds.html.

212. Body For Life, http://bodyforlife.com/.

213. 10 Movements Your Joints Will Love, Kelli Russell, ERYT/BY, October 29, 2015, http://www.kellirussell.com/10-movements-your-joints-will-love/.

214. Hans F. Hansen, Quotes, http://www.goodreads.com/quotes/1045653-it-takes-nothing-to-join-the-crowd-it-takes-everything-to.

215. 31 Natural Pest Control Methods For Those Little Things That Really Bug You! http://www.maryannsawyers.com/Blog/Archive?tag=Natural Remedies.

216. Sunny Days, Keeping Those Clouds Away, John McDougall MD, May, 2005, https://www.drmcdougall.com/misc/2005nl/may/050500pusunshine.htm.

217. 11 Surprising Health Benefits Of Sleep, Alyssa Sparacino, http://www.health.com/health/gallery/0,,20459221_2,00.html.

218. Meet the Physician-Farmer Who Grows The Plants He Prescribes To His Patients, Naomi Imatome-Yun, June 27, 2016, http://www.forksoverknives.com/meet-physician-farmer-grows-plants-prescribes-patients/.

219. Mammograms Cause Breast Cancer, Dr. Ben Johnson, https://m.youtube.com/watch?v=3MCKNxYCUpM.

220. Early Detection For Cancer Is A Risky Business, John McDougall MD, August 2014, https://www.drmcdougall.com/misc/2014nl/aug/early.htm.

221. Recommendations For Primary Care, U.S. Preventive Services Task Force, http://www.uspreventiveservicestaskforce.org/Page/Name/recommendations.

222. Published Recommendations, U.S. Preventive Services Task Force, http://www.uspreventiveservicestaskforce.org/BrowseRec/Index/browse-recommendations.

223. Cochrane, Trusted Evidence, Informed Decisions, Better Health, http://www.cochrane.org/about-us.

224. About The USPSTF, (U.S. Preventive Services Task Force), http://www.uspreventiveservicestaskforce.org/Page/Name/about-the-uspstf.

225. Mammography Screening: Truth, Lies and Controversy, Peter Gotzsche, MD, https://www.drmcdougall.com/misc/2012nl/may/mammography.htm.

226. Back To Eden Official Film, 2011, https://vimeo.com/28055108.

227. How To Get Back To The Garden of Eden, http://www.backto-edenfilm.com/how-to-grow-an-organic-garden.html.

228. Eat, Pray, Love, Sony Pictures, http://www.sonypictures.com/movies/eatpraylove/.

229. Full Catastrophe Living: Using The Wisdom Of Your Body And Mind To face Stress, Pain And Illness, Jon Kabat-Zinn, http://www.goodreads.com/book/show/589455.Full_Catastrophe_Living.

230. Balanced You by Jenny Harkleroad, www.BalancedYou.org.

231. Feeling Good Together: The Secret To Making Troubled Relationships Work, http://www.goodreads.com/book/show/5680626-feeling-good-together?ac=1&from_search=true.

232. Audible, www.audible.com.

233. The Doctrine and Covenants, Section 89, Joseph Smith, February 27, 1833, https://www.lds.org/scriptures/dc-testament/dc/89?lang=eng.

234. The Starch Solution, John A. McDougall, MD, 2012.

235. The China Study by T. Colin Campbell, PhD & Thomas M. Campbell II, 2006.

236. Prevent and Reverse Heart Disease, Caldwell Esselstyn Jr. M.D., 2007.

237. Balanced You by Jenny Harkleroad, www.BalancedYou.org.

238. Emotional Eating vs. Mindful Eating, Tips To Help You Fight Food Cravings And Satisfy Your Needs With Mindful Eating, http://www.helpguide.org/articles/diet-weight-loss/emotional-eating.htm.

239. Discovering The Word of Wisdom, Jane Birch, 2013.

240. Whole Food, Plant-Based (WFPB) Made Easy, Jane Birch, http://discoveringthewordofwisdom.com/wfpb-made-easy/.

241. The Happy Herbivore, Lindsay S. Nixon, 2015, https://www.amazon.com/Happy-Herbivore-Guide-Plant-Based-Living/dp/1941631002/.

242. PlantPure Jumpstart, http://shop.plantpurenation.com/what-is-a-jumpstart.php.

243. Happy Herbivore: 7-day Meal Plans, https://www.getmealplans.com/.

244. Help! I'm NOT Enjoying My New Food, Jane Birch, Dr. McDougall's Online Discussion Board, https://www.drmcdougall.com/forums/viewtopic.php?f=14&t=2454.

245. Chef Brad's WonderFlour, http://chefbrad.com/2016/06/chef-brads-wonderflour/.

246. http://chefbrad.com/2016/06/chef-brads-wonderflour/.

Made in the USA
Charleston, SC
17 January 2017